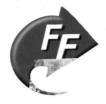

THE LIBRARY
THE LEARNING AND DEVELO'
THE CAL...DALE ROYAL HO
HALIFAX   W

Fast Facts:
Chronic Pain

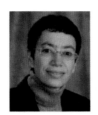

M Soledad Cepeda MD PhD

Professor (Designate)
Department of Anesthesia
Tufts–New England Medical Center and
Tufts University School of Medicine
Boston, Massachusetts, USA

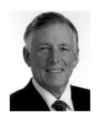

Michael J Cousins AM MD FFPMANZCA

Head of Anaesthesia and Pain Management
Department of Anaesthesia
Royal North Shore Hospital
University of Sydney
New South Wales, Australia

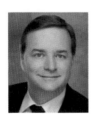

Daniel B Carr MD FABPM FFPMANZCA(Hon)

Saltonstall Professor of Pain Research
Departments of Anesthesia and Medicine
Tufts–New England Medical Center and
Tufts University School of Medicine
Boston, Massachusetts, USA
Chief Executive Officer and Chief Medical Officer
Javelin Pharmaceuticals Inc.
Cambridge, Massachusetts, USA

Declaration of Independence
This book is as balanced and as practical as we can make it.
Ideas for improvement are always welcome:

Calderdale and Huddersfield NHS Trust

B60565

HEALTH PRESS

Fast Facts: Chronic Pain
First published January 2007

Text © 2007 M Soledad Cepeda, Michael J Cousins, Daniel B Carr
© 2007 in this edition Health Press Limited
Health Press Limited, Elizabeth House, Queen Street, Abingdon,
Oxford OX14 3LN, UK
Tel: +44 (0)1235 523233
Fax: +44 (0)1235 523238

Book orders can be placed by telephone or via the website.
For regional distributors or to order via the website, please go to:
www.fastfacts.com
For telephone orders, please call 01752 202301 (UK), +44 1752 202301 (Europe),
1 800 247 6553 (USA, toll free) or +1 419 281 1802 (Americas).

Fast Facts is a trademark of Health Press Limited.

All rights reserved. No part of this publication may be reproduced, stored in a
retrieval system, or transmitted in any form or by any means, electronic, mechanical,
photocopying, recording or otherwise, without the express permission of the
publisher.

The rights of M Soledad Cepeda, Michael J Cousins and Daniel B Carr to be
identified as the authors of this work have been asserted in accordance with the
Copyright, Designs & Patents Act 1988 Sections 77 and 78.

The publisher and the authors have made every effort to ensure the accuracy of this
book, but cannot accept responsibility for any errors or omissions.

For all drugs, please consult the product labeling approved in your country for
prescribing information.

Registered names, trademarks, etc. used in this book, even when not marked as such,
are not to be considered unprotected by law.

A CIP record for this title is available from the British Library.

ISBN 978-1-903734-87-2

Cepeda MS (M Soledad)
Fast Facts: Chronic Pain/
M Soledad Cepeda, Michael J Cousins, Daniel B Carr

Medical illustrations by Annamaria Dutto, Withernsea, UK.
Typesetting and page layout by Zed, Oxford, UK.
Printed by Fine Print (Services) Ltd, Oxford, UK.

Text printed with vegetable inks on fully biodegradable and
recyclable paper manufactured from sustainable forests.

444   001

Low emissions
during production

Low   Sustainable
chlorine   forests

THE LIBRARY
LEARNING AND DEVELOPMENT CENTRE
The CALDERDALE ROYAL HOSPITAL
HALIFAX HX3 0PW

Glossary of abbreviations

AMPA receptor: α-amino-3-hydroxy-5-methyl-4-isoxazole propionic acid receptor; an ionotropic transmembrane receptor for glutamate that mediates fast synaptic transmission in the central nervous system

ARS: adjective rating scale

CGRP: calcitonin gene-related peptide; a peptide with a different action from calcitonin – it has no effect on calcium metabolism but is a strong vasodilator

COX-2 inhibitor: cyclooxygenase-2 inhibitor; a subtype of non-steroidal anti-inflammatory drug that preferentially inhibits the isoform of cyclooxygenase, COX-2, which is expressed during inflammation

DMARD: disease-modifying antirheumatic drug

DREZ: dorsal root entry zone; *see* 'Substantia gelatinosa' (page 6)

HRQoL: health-related quality of life

NK1 receptor: neurokinin 1 receptor; the receptor for substance P

NMDA receptor: N-methyl D-aspartate receptor; an ionotropic receptor for glutamate. Activation of NMDA receptors results in an influx of Ca^{++}, which plays a critical role in synaptic plasticity

NRS: numeric rating scale

NSAID: non-steroidal anti-inflammatory drug; aspirin-like drug that reduces pain and inflammation arising from injured tissue

PKC: protein kinase C; isozyme present in numerous tissues that catalyzes the phosphorylation of intracellular proteins, altering their activities. The enzymes are activated by agents that cause increases in intracellular calcium and cleavage of phosphoinositides

TOPS: Treatment Outcomes in Pain Survey

VAS: visual analog scale

Glossary

Addiction (psychological dependence): pattern of compulsive drug use characterized by a continued craving for a substance (e.g. an opioid) and the need to use that substance for effects other than pain relief

Adjuvant analgesic drug: a drug that is not a primary analgesic but that has independent or additive analgesic properties

Algogenic: producing pain

Allodynia: condition in which ordinarily non-painful stimuli evoke pain

Analgesia: the relief of pain by pharmacological or non-pharmacological interventions, or by endogenous processes

Breakthrough pain: intermittent, transient exacerbation of pain that can occur spontaneously or in relation to a specific activity

Cauda equina: a bundle of nerves, resembling the tail of a horse, that descends vertically from the lumbar, sacral and coccygeal spinal nerves

Dyspareunia: difficult or painful sexual intercourse

Epidural: situated within the spinal canal, on or outside the dura mater (the tough membrane surrounding the spinal cord); synonyms are 'extradural' and 'peridural'

Ligamentum flavum: the strong ligament that connects the laminae of the vertebrae; it protects the nerves and spinal cord, and stabilizes the spine so that excessive motion between the vertebral bodies does not occur

Meta-analysis: combining the results of several related studies to obtain more reliable conclusions

Mixed opioid agonist–antagonist: a compound that has an affinity for two or more types of opioid receptor, and blocks opioid effects on one receptor type while producing opioid effects on a second receptor type

Neuropathic pain: pain that arises from damage to the central or peripheral nervous systems

Nitric oxide: a gas that acts in many tissues to regulate a diverse range of physiological processes

Nociception: the process of pain transmission; usually relating to a receptive neuron for painful sensations

Nociceptor: nerve ending responsible for nociception

Opioid agonist: any morphine-like compound that produces bodily effects, including pain relief, sedation, constipation and respiratory depression

Opioid partial agonist: a compound that has an affinity for and stimulates physiological activity at the same cell receptors as opioid agonists but that produces only a partial (i.e. submaximal) bodily response

Pain: an unpleasant sensory and emotional experience associated with actual or potential tissue damage or described in terms of such damage

Peridural: synonym for epidural and extradural

Physical dependence: physiological adaptation of the body to the presence of a drug, which manifests as the need to continue dosing in order to avoid precipitation of an abstinence syndrome

Prostaglandin: chemical that produces pain, inflammation and central sensitization

Psychological dependence: *see* 'Addiction'

Substance P: a neuropeptide belonging to the tachykinin family that functions as a neurotransmitter

Substantia gelatinosa: a narrow, dense column of small neurons at the most superficial extension of the dorsal gray matter that runs the length of the spinal cord

Tolerance: a common physiological response to chronic use of opioids and other selected medications, such that progressively higher doses are required to maintain the effect (e.g. analgesia) produced by the initial dose

Introduction

All clinicians, regardless of specialty, will see patients with pain that has persisted for more than 6 months. It is now clear that persistent pain is a disease entity with a broad range of physical and psychological pathologies involving the peripheral and central nervous systems. Its costs as a disease per se are substantial across every segment of society.

Chronic pain is not tabulated as a separate diagnosis in the World Health Organization's comprehensive estimates of global health burdens associated with highly prevalent conditions. Yet it is through chronic pain that many of the greatest global health burdens – cancer, HIV/AIDS, diabetes, arthritis, alcoholism and trauma (including war) – exact their long-term human, social and economic toll. Mental health problems such as anxiety and depression also place sufferers at increased risk of developing chronic pain, while those with chronic pain are prone to develop new anxiety or depression.

Pain, which has long been of little concern in healthcare, has now taken center stage because of consumer demands for enhanced quality of life. As a consequence, new standards have been introduced that require its routine assessment and control. In much of the world, the relief of pain is now viewed as a human right – a point of view that is spreading.

Fast Facts: Chronic Pain summarizes the key facts about chronic pain for busy frontline practitioners. We describe a variety of chronic pain syndromes, discuss their pathogenesis and treatment(s), and provide the evidence for treatment efficacy.

This handbook seeks to distill a great deal of pain-related evidence, much of which cannot be synthesized mathematically because of the poor quality of many pain trials and the wide range of outcomes assessed across trials. Therefore, we have not attempted to tabulate the specific evidence supporting each therapeutic intervention, but have adopted the current practice in clinical decision-making of using clinical trial literature as 'tools not rules' and to practice 'evidence-guided' rather than 'evidence-based' medicine.

Acknowledgments. As clinicians and teachers we recognize the multidisciplinary and interdisciplinary nature of chronic pain and those who treat it. This book is dedicated to our families, in grateful acknowledgment of their support during our often long hours; our colleagues, who have shared and thereby lightened our own professional burdens; and our patients and their families, who have sought to reclaim lives taken from them by chronic pain.

In addition, the Saltonstall Fund for Pain Research has generously supported this and many other research and educational activities of Drs Cepeda and Carr.

Mechanisms and definitions

Defining pain

There are many ways to classify pain; for example, by duration, etiology or intensity (Table 1.1). As understanding of the cellular mechanisms of pain has increased, proposals have been advanced to classify pain according to the predominant pathophysiological mechanism thought to be involved.

Present-day pain research was heralded by the publication of Melzack's and Wall's 'gate control theory' in 1965, which provided a model for the modulation of incoming nociceptive information by the central nervous system (CNS). After publication of that model, researchers never again viewed the peripheral nervous system (PNS) or CNS as collections of cables passively transmitting nociceptive information.

TABLE 1.1

Possible pain classifications

Duration	Probable mechanism
• Acute	• Inflammation
• Subacute	• Central sensitization
• Chronic	• Sprouting of mechanoreceptive fibers in the dorsal horn
Etiology	• Sprouting of noradrenergic axons around sensory neurons at dorsal root ganglia
• Cancerous	
• Ischemic	• Pathological cross-talk between novel connections across previously separate pathways
• Postoperative	
Intensity	**Type of injured tissue**
• Mild	• Nociceptive
• Moderate	• Neuropathic
• Severe	• Visceral
	• Somatic

The nervous system is dynamic; it is 'plastic' in that its structure and function are shaped and reshaped by activity within it, and at each level it continually amplifies or inhibits the signals that the brain ultimately interprets as pain. This plasticity is fundamental to the understanding of both the perpetuation of pain in some pain syndromes and the mechanisms of action of pain treatment modalities.

Mechanisms of pain

A stimulus of intensity sufficient to threaten tissue damage activates specialized nerve endings termed nociceptors. The cell bodies of these nociceptors (first-order neurons) are located outside the spinal cord in the dorsal root ganglia and extend their dendritic processes to the periphery. Activation of nociceptors triggers a volley of incoming impulses that travel to the spinal cord along both myelinated (Aδ) and unmyelinated (C) nerve fibers. These fibers enter the spinal cord almost exclusively through the dorsal root, and synapse in the dorsal horn of the spinal cord, where they project to higher levels such as the thalamus, hypothalamus, reticular system and cortex of the brain (Figure 1.1).

Roughly speaking, the higher-level sites bring about the aversive emotional feelings (thalamus and limbic system), alterations in sleep pattern (reticular system and hypothalamus) and stress responses (hypothalamus) that pain may evoke.

The PNS and CNS do not passively transduce stimuli and convey sensory information. Instead, painful stimuli trigger biological processes that then amplify or inhibit the pain signal.

Potentiation. After tissue or nerve damage, peripheral nociceptors become sensitized to noxious stimuli owing to the formation and accumulation of algogenic and inflammatory mediators in the periphery, such as prostanoids, interleukins, bradykinin and histamine. Peripheral sensitization and heightened afferent activity in pain fibers elicit functional, chemical and anatomic reorganization in spinal cord neurons. These changes lead to long-term central potentiation, a form of pain memory characterized by progressively enhanced and prolonged spinal neuronal responses to afferent impulses.

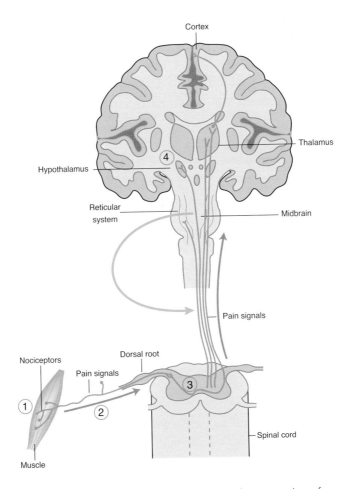

Figure 1.1 The pathways of pain. (1) Transduction: the conversion of a noxious stimulus into electrical energy by a peripheral nociceptor. (2) Transmission: propagation of the signal through the peripheral nervous system via first-order neurons. (3) Modulation: adjustment of pain intensity at the point where first-order neurons synapse with second-order neurons in the dorsal horn of the spinal cord. (4) Perception: the cerebral cortical response to nociceptive signals projected to the brain by third-order neurons. Stimulation of the descending pathway from the brain (green arrow) sends inhibitory responses back to the periphery – the brain can order the release of chemicals with an analgesic effect that may reduce or even abolish some forms of pain.

This spatially and temporally exaggerated processing of persistent nociceptive information translates clinically into sensations of pain, not only in the injured tissue (primary hyperalgesia), but also in surrounding uninjured tissue (secondary hyperalgesia), with repetitive stimulation producing progressively greater neuronal responses.

Central potentiation is due to the release by efferent nociceptive neurons of excitatory mediators such as substance P and glutamate that bind to neurokinin 1 (NK1) and N-methyl D-aspartate (NMDA) receptors, respectively, in the dorsal horn. Concurrent activation of these receptors allows a massive influx of calcium into second-order neurons, the cell bodies of which lie within the dorsal horn of the spinal cord. Consequently, calcium-dependent intracellular enzymes such as protein kinase C (PKC) are activated, which catalyze the production of nitric oxide and prostaglandins. These protein kinases also activate other proteins such as ion channels or enzymes (Figure 1.2).

Inhibition. Pain also triggers processes that dampen the perception of nociceptive stimuli. Nociceptive afferent traffic ascends to the midbrain and brainstem, where it activates descending pathways that inhibit spinal pain transmission. These descending inhibitory systems are stimulated by endogenous opioids, as well as monoamines such as norepinephrine (noradrenaline) and serotonin. These systems inhibit spinal nociceptive transmission through the local release of inhibitory transmitters such as γ-aminobutyric acid (GABA), glycine, adenosine and endogenous opioids at the spinal level. Analgesics such as opioids and tricyclic antidepressants, in addition to their other mechanisms of action, activate these inhibitory systems. Furthermore, pain elicits a stress hormone response that includes the systemic secretion of endogenous opioids from the anterior pituitary and the adrenal medulla.

Interpretation

Pain is more than the nociceptive cascade described above. Pain is 'an unpleasant sensory and emotional experience associated with actual or potential tissue damage, or described in terms of such damage'. Because it is an experience, pain itself cannot be measured directly. Pain, like consciousness itself, is constructed by complex brain processes that

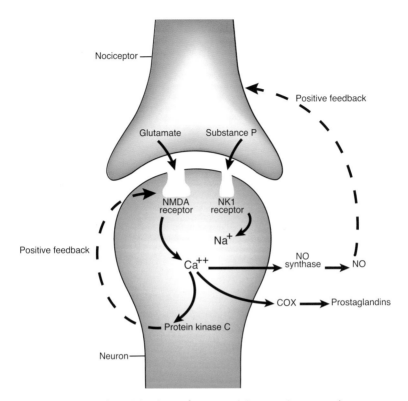

Figure 1.2 Central sensitization. After nerve injury, nociceptors release excitatory mediators such as substance P and glutamate, which bind to neurokinin 1 (NK1) and N-methyl D-aspartate (NMDA) receptors, respectively, in the dorsal horn. This results in an increase in intracellular calcium concentration and subsequent intracellular activation of the calcium-dependent enzyme protein kinase C (PKC). PKC catalyzes the production of nitric oxide (NO). NO and PKC enhance postsynaptic neuronal excitability by increasing the efficacy of receptor ion channel complexes. The influx of calcium also results in the production of superoxide from mitochondria, with potential cell dysfunction and cell death if intracellular calcium stores are markedly increased for prolonged intervals. COX, cyclooxygenase.

are strongly affected by a person's attitudes, beliefs, personality and interpretation of the significance of nociceptive stimuli. Central to the understanding of clinical pain is the concept that pain may be present without an obvious source or cause.

Mechanisms of neuropathic pain

Definition. Neuropathic pain is initiated or caused by a primary lesion of the PNS or CNS. Patients often complain not only of spontaneous pain, but also of pain from stimuli that are not normally painful (allodynia). For example, a light touch may be described as painful. Important types of neuropathic pain and their probable causes are shown in Table 1.2, and are discussed in more detail in subsequent chapters.

Pathophysiology. A variety of neuropathic pain syndromes share overlapping pathogenic mechanisms. Those pain syndromes that have unique pathogenic mechanisms are discussed in the relevant chapters. Among other classifications, pathogenic mechanisms can be considered as either peripheral or central.

Peripheral nerve injury produces axonal membrane hyperexcitability that leads to spontaneous generation of ectopic impulses. In addition, changes in the chemical environment surrounding the damaged axon trigger ectopic nerve action potentials, which lead to further impulses (Figure 1.3). Abnormal repetitive firing of injured axons occurs because of the accumulation of sodium channels at the site of injury, which creates a lower threshold for the initiation of action potentials (Figure 1.4). Aβ fibers rather than C fibers show the greatest degree of

TABLE 1.2

Types of neuropathic pain and their probable causes

Type	Cause
Trigeminal neuralgia	Compression of trigeminal ganglion or its branches
Postherpetic neuralgia	Shingles
Complex regional pain syndrome	Trauma/surgery/inflammation
Diabetic neuropathy	Persistent hyperglycemia (diabetes)
Central pain	Trauma to the spinal cord; stroke
Phantom pain	Amputation
Postincisional pain	Surgery

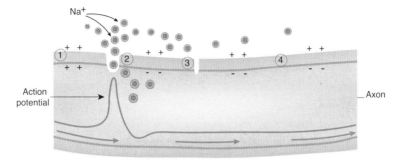

Figure 1.3 Cross-section of an axon, with an action potential (AP) moving from left to right. (1) The AP has passed, the sodium channels are inactivated and the membrane is hyperpolarized. (2) As an impulse passes along the axon the membrane becomes depolarized; at the peak of the AP the sodium channels open and Na⁺ ions flow into the axon. (3) Na⁺ ions move in from the adjacent region and depolarize the membrane such that the sodium channels start to open. (4) When the nerve is not transmitting an impulse, a resting potential is maintained across the polarized membrane, with the inside of the axon being negative with respect to the outside.

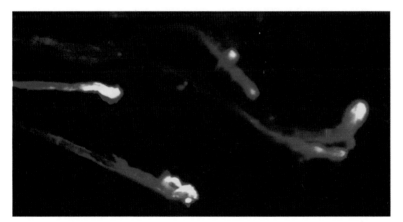

Figure 1.4 Immunofluorescence labeling showing accumulation of sodium channels on the membrane of an axon in a chronic neuroma. Note the intense labeling of the end bulb, which indicates an increased density and number of sodium channels in the neuroma. This abnormal concentration of sodium channels leads to abnormally persistent repetitive firing of injured nerves. Photograph provided courtesy of Dr Marshall Devor.

spontaneous ectopic discharge after peripheral nerve injury. Aβ fibers are specialized for light touch and are therefore likely to mediate the allodynia experienced after nerve injury. Nerve injury also triggers the production of a series of inflammatory mediators that promote ectopic activity in primary afferent fibers. These mediators are produced by macrophages that migrate to sites of nerve injury and contribute to chronic inflammation in their immediate environment.

Central nerve injury. The generation of ectopic impulses is not limited to injured axons; neurons of the dorsal root ganglia whose peripheral axons have been damaged also exhibit spontaneous activity. Following nerve injury, sympathetic fibers may sprout and form 'baskets' around dorsal root ganglia cell bodies; at the same time α_2 receptors are expressed on neurons of the dorsal root ganglia. These changes allow for activation of the neurons via sympathetic fibers.

Central nerve injury activates NMDA and α-amino-3-hydroxy-5-methyl-4-isoxazole propionic acid (AMPA) receptors. This leads to an increase in intracellular calcium concentration and subsequent intracellular activation of PKC and nitric oxide synthase with production of nitric oxide. Nitric oxide and PKC enhance postsynaptic neuronal excitability by increasing the efficacy of receptor ion-channel complexes in the postsynaptic membrane. In addition to the activation of NMDA receptors, spinal cord hyperexcitability could be produced by upregulation of sodium channels and voltage-sensitive calcium channels in neurons of the dorsal root ganglia.

The sensitization (increased excitability) and increased synaptic efficacy of second-order neurons termed 'wide dynamic range neurons' (i.e. neurons that respond to a range of noxious and non-noxious stimuli) could explain the allodynia that patients experience after nerve injury. The central hyperexcitable state and enlargement of the area in the periphery where stimulation evokes a neuronal response are sustained by ectopic peripheral nerve activity that causes ongoing release of neurotransmitters in the spinal cord (see Figure 1.2).

Reorganization of neurons. After nerve injury a variety of neuronal growth factors are released; these can produce long-term modifications in neuronal phenotype and in the structural organization of synaptic connectivity through their ability to potentiate over the long term.

Key points – mechanisms and definitions

- The nervous system is dynamic and plastic; painful stimuli trigger biological processes that lead to amplification or inhibition of the pain signal.
- Nociceptive input activates descending pathways that inhibit spinal pain transmission. These descending pathways are potential targets for analgesic drugs.
- Neuropathic pain is produced by a lesion of the peripheral or central nervous system.
- Nerve injury produces hyperexcitability and spontaneous generation of ectopic impulses in axons and neurons.
- Ectopic peripheral nerve activity contributes to the central hyperexcitable state and the enlargement of neuronal receptive fields.
- After nerve injury there is also a loss of spinal inhibitory control.

Aβ fibers develop abnormal connections with the nociceptive neurons of the dorsal horn. This structural reorganization may underlie the increased sensitivity to normally innocuous mechanical stimulation after nerve injury.

In addition, nerve injury triggers glial activation. Glial cells release proinflammatory cytokines (tumor necrosis factor, interleukin-1, interleukin-6) and brain-derived neurotrophic factor. These substances, both individually and in concert, contribute to the central hyperexcitability by directly activating neurons.

Loss of inhibition. Moreover, after nerve injury there is also a loss of spinal inhibitory control. After the influx of calcium associated with nerve injury, mitochondrial superoxide is produced, which leads to cell dysfunction and death of interneurons with inhibitory control. The death of these neurons could explain the decrease in immunoreactivity for GABA, an inhibitory transmitter, in the dorsal horn of the spinal cord after nerve damage.

Finally, the persistent afferent input after peripheral nerve injury provokes changes in the nerve structure of the rostroventromedial medulla. These changes in turn encourage tonic discharge (firing at regular intervals) of the descending pathways that facilitate nociceptive transmission, further perpetuating the hyperexcitable state observed after nerve injury.

Key references

Baron R. Peripheral neuropathic pain: from mechanisms to symptoms. *Clin J Pain* 2000(2 suppl);16:S12–20.

Cepeda MS, Carr DB. Overview of pain management. In: *Approaches to Pain Management. An Essential Guide for Clinical Leaders.* Oakbrook Terrace, Illinois: Joint Commission Resources, 2003:1–20.

Chung JM, Dib-Hajj SD, Lawson SN. Sodium channel subtypes and neuropathic pain. In: Dostrovsky JO, Carr DB, Koltzenburg M, eds. *Proceedings of the 10th World Congress on Pain.* Seattle: IASP Press, 2003:99–114.

Devor M. Neuropathic pain: what do we do with all these theories? *Acta Anaesthesiol Scand* 2001;45:1121–7.

Dickenson AH, Matthews EA, Suzuki E. Central nervous system mechanisms of pain in peripheral neuropathy. In: Hansson PT, Fields HL, Hill RG, Marchettini P, eds. *Neuropathic Pain: Pathophysiology and Treatment.* Seattle: IASP Press, 2001:85–106.

Eidelman A, Carr DB. Taxonomy of cancer pain. In: de Leon-Casasola OA, ed. *Cancer Pain: Pharmacological, Interventional and Palliative Care Approaches.* Philadelphia: WB Saunders, 2006:3–12.

Ji RR, Woolf CJ. Neuronal plasticity and signal transduction in nociceptive neurons: implications for the initiation and maintenance of pathological pain. *Neurobiol Dis* 2001;8:1–10.

Mayer DJ, Mao J, Holt J, Price DD. Cellular mechanisms of neuropathic pain, morphine tolerance, and their interactions. *Proc Natl Acad Sci USA* 1999;96:7731–6.

Melzack R, Wall PD. Pain mechanisms: a new theory. *Science* 1965;150:171–9.

Watkins LR, Maier SF. Beyond neurons: evidence that immune and glial cells contribute to pathological pain states. *Physiol Rev* 2002;82: 981–1011.

Woolf CJ, Bennett GJ, Doherty M et al. Towards a mechanism-based classification of pain. *Pain* 1998;77: 227–9.

The initial evaluation of a patient's pain forms the foundation for a rational treatment plan and must therefore be as thorough as possible. For patients with chronic pain this evaluation should include:

- a detailed history
- a physical examination (with particular attention being paid to neurological function)
- a psychosocial assessment
- diagnostic testing (e.g. imaging) when appropriate.

Clearly, the history, physical examination and any laboratory evaluation performed to assess chronic pain may overlap with those carried out for general medical diagnosis and therapy.

Many patients with pain due to cancer or other serious illnesses such as HIV/AIDS experience pain from multiple mechanisms, locations and etiologies. These patients may simultaneously experience acute and chronic pain; somatic and neuropathic pain related to the primary diagnosis or its treatment; or pain from unrelated, possibly pre-existing, medical conditions. Because of the multiple and evolving etiologies of pain, each time a clinician assesses a patient at risk of undertreated pain a fresh evaluation of pain must be made. Unless pain is assessed systematically and classified according to its likely origin, then the patient is at risk of receiving suboptimal treatment. Even after an initial pain treatment plan is put in place, the source and severity of a person's pain and the effectiveness of treatment may fluctuate, and therefore should be reviewed and documented at regular intervals.

History

The patient's pain history should document the location, duration, type and intensity of the pain, any exacerbating or alleviating factors, previous treatments and response to them, and the meaning of the pain to the patient and their family (Table 2.1).

The patient's self-report is a more accurate assessment of pain than are vital signs, outward behavior or observer estimates; however, the last

TABLE 2.1

Questions to ask when documenting the patient's pain history

Dimension	Question
Location	Where is your pain?
Onset	When did your pain start?
Variation	Has the intensity of the pain changed?
Frequency	How often does the pain occur?
Intensity	How much does it hurt now? How much does it hurt at its worst? How much does it hurt at its best? (for scales, see Figure 2.2, page 22)
Characteristic/type	How would you describe your pain? (e.g. burning, shooting, throbbing)
Aggravating factors	What makes your pain worse?
Relieving factors	What makes your pain better?
Impairment	How much does the pain affect your daily activities? How much does the pain affect your social life? Have you had changes in mood as a result of the pain?
Previous treatments	What treatments have you tried to relieve the pain?
Response to treatment	What treatments have been effective?
Meaning of the pain	What do you think is the cause of your pain?

is, by default, important in neonates, infants and individuals of any age with severe cognitive impairment or poor language skills. To avoid underestimating pain in individuals with poor cognition or in those incapable of communicating, indirect indices of pain such as facial expression or body language become more important.

Pain location. It is helpful to ask patients to identify on a body map the areas where they experience pain (Figure 2.1). Body pain maps help clinicians to assess pain and monitor treatment efficacy.

Patient Name: _____

Date: _____

Clinician Name: _____

1. Indicate (in blue ink) on the figures below area(s) of consistent pain.

2. Indicate (in red ink) on the figures below area(s) of intermittent chronic pain.

3. Indicate level of pain on the scale below.

0   1   2   3   4   5   6   7   8   9   10

no pain   worst imaginable pain

4. Describe how the above indicated pain affects your functioning: _____

_____

_____

_____

5. Other: _____

Clinician: _____

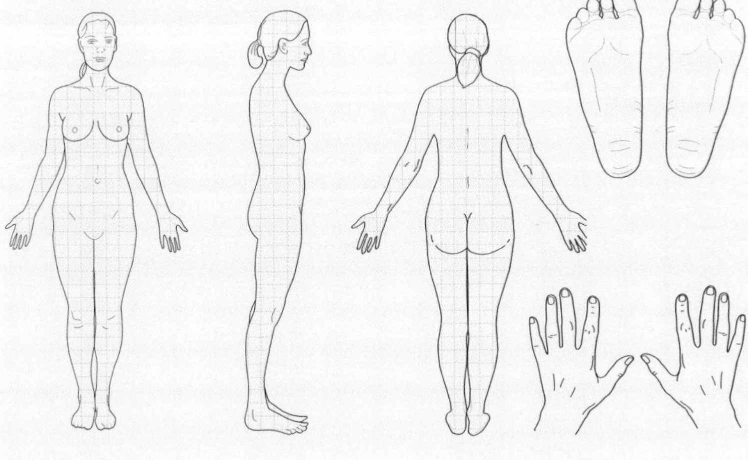

Figure 2.1 Pain assessment form, including a body map, which can be used to document pain symptoms such as location and intensity.

Pain intensity is the most frequently evaluated dimension of pain. During the titration of analgesics for acute time-limited pain of obvious cause (e.g. dental extraction) it may suffice to monitor only pain intensity and forego tracking other aspects of the multidimensional pain experience.

21

Assessment tools. Three types of assessment tool are commonly used to quantify pain intensity (Figure 2.2):

- visual analog scale (VAS)
- numeric rating scale (NRS)
- adjective rating scale (ARS).

The visual analog scale is presented graphically with a 10-cm baseline and endpoint descriptors. Patients place a mark on the line at a point that best represents their pain. Their responses are scored by measuring the distance of the mark from the left-hand end of the scale ('anchor').

The numeric rating scale may be presented graphically or verbally, with 0 representing 'no pain' and 10 representing 'the worst possible pain'. Patients volunteer a number that best represents their pain intensity.

The adjective rating scale employs descriptors of pain intensity such as 'none', 'mild', 'moderate' or 'severe'.

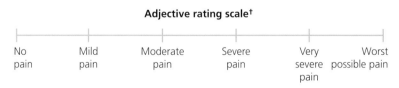

Visual analog scale (VAS)*

No pain — Pain as bad as it could possibly be

Numeric rating scale†

0 1 2 3 4 5 6 7 8 9 10

No pain — Moderate pain — Worst possible pain

Adjective rating scale†

No pain — Mild pain — Moderate pain — Severe pain — Very severe pain — Worst possible pain

*A 10-cm baseline is recommended for VAS scales.
†If used as a graphic rating scale, a 10-cm baseline is recommended.

Figure 2.2 Pain intensity scales.

Patient's perception. We now know that patients regard a decrement in pain intensity in relation to the baseline (pretreatment) pain intensity. The more severe the baseline pain, the greater the decrement in VAS or NRS score needed to achieve clinical importance for the patient.

Neurological examination

In patients with chronic pain it is essential to perform a comprehensive neurological examination in addition to a routine physical assessment. The neurological examination should evaluate:

- mental status
- motor system
- sensory perception
- deep tendon reflex
- cranial nerve function.

Mental status. An evaluation of mental status should assess the patient's level of alertness; degree of orientation with respect to time, place and person; general appearance; behavior and mood; and intellectual function including comprehension, ability to pay attention, insight and memory. The patient may be asked to remember several objects mentioned earlier in the course of the examination, to repeat sentences, to solve simple mathematical problems or to carry out commands of graded complexity.

Motor system. An evaluation of motor system should check the appearance of the muscles (e.g. atrophy), their tone (e.g. flaccid) and strength. Observation of gait can provide information on muscle strength; any indication of impaired vestibular, cerebellar or dorsal column function should be documented. Latent weakness can be detected by asking patients to walk on their toes and heels. Heel walking is the most sensitive bedside test for weakness of foot dorsiflexion, while toe walking is the best way to detect early weakness of foot plantar flexion.

Muscle atrophy can be documented by circumferential measurements of the extremities (e.g. the calf and thigh bilaterally). A difference of 2 cm or more at the same level is indicative of atrophy.

Sensory perception can be evaluated with different types of stimuli, such as light touch, painful squeeze or pinprick, temperature and pressure/vibration. A freshly opened alcohol wipe may be used as a bedside probe of deficits in cold perception, or to elicit cold allodynia.

Deep tendon reflex testing is the most objective part of the neurological examination, since the reflexes are not under voluntary control and testing does not depend on the patient's cooperation. Alterations in reflexes are often early signs of neurological dysfunction.

Cranial nerve function. The 12 cranial nerves relay messages between the brain and the head and neck. They mediate motor and sensory functions, including vision, smell, and movement of the tongue and vocal cords. The evaluation of the fifth cranial nerve (affected in trigeminal neuralgia, see Chapter 3) requires the assessment of facial sensation, jaw strength and movement, and corneal reflexes.

Psychosocial assessment

The psychosocial assessment should explore the patient's:
- mood
- coping skills
- family support structure
- signs and symptoms of anxiety or depression
- expectations regarding pain management.

Persistent pain commonly undermines mood, vitality, function and other dimensions of health-related quality of life (HRQoL). Thus, it is important to monitor how pain and its treatment affect function, daily activities, mood, sleep patterns and other aspects of HRQoL.

Quality-of-life questionnaires specifically designed for patients with chronic non-malignant pain have been developed in an effort to better gauge how pain and pain treatments affect HRQoL. For example, the Treatment Outcomes in Pain Survey (TOPS) questionnaire (Table 2.2) incorporates 61 items of the Multidimensional Pain Inventory, ten items of the Oswestry Disability Questionnaire and six items of the Medical Outcome Study. It is a well-validated tool in patients with chronic pain.

TABLE 2.2

Example questions taken from the Treatment Outcomes in Pain Survey

1. The following items concern activities you might perform during a typical day. Does your health now limit you in these activities? If so, by how much?

	Not at all	A little	A lot
Vigorous activities (e.g. running, lifting heavy objects, participating in strenuous sports)			
Moderate activities (e.g. moving a table, pushing a vacuum cleaner, bowling or playing golf)			
Climbing several flights of stairs			
Climbing one flight of stairs			
Bending, kneeling or stooping			
Walking more than a mile			
Walking several blocks			
Walking one block			
Bathing or dressing yourself			
Combing your hair			
Writing			
Talking			

2. During the *past 4 weeks*, to what extent has your physical health or emotional problems interfered with your normal social activities with family, friends, neighbors or groups?

Not at all   Slightly   Moderately   Quite a bit   Extremely

3. How much does your pain get in the way of:

	Not at all	A little	Moderately	Quite a lot	A lot
Enjoying your social activities or hobbies?					
Doing any social activities or hobbies?					
Getting along with your husband/wife/ significant other/family?					
Getting along with friends outside of your family?					
The pleasure you get from being with your family?					
How well you can plan things?					

Diagnostic tests

Imaging tests help physicians to confirm or rule out diagnoses suggested by findings in the medical history or physical examination. Radiographs provide details of bone structure, while bone scans are performed to rule out occult fractures (small fractures not visible on routine radiographs) or inflammatory processes (such as infection or certain tumors). Bone scans also help determine whether a compression fracture of the vertebral body is old or new, as an old fracture will not 'light up', but a new one will; however, they cannot differentiate between tumor, infection or fracture with adjoining inflammation. In such cases, computed tomography (CT) or magnetic resonance imaging (MRI) can better characterize the lesion. Similarly, in patients whose findings suggest nerve impairment, CT or MRI can help define an anatomic cause.

Key points – assessment of pain

- A thorough evaluation of pain is the foundation for a rational treatment plan.
- Persistent pain is a disease entity per se that can undermine many dimensions of health-related quality of life.
- The patient's pain history should document the location, duration, type (character) and intensity of pain, exacerbating or alleviating factors, previous treatments and response to them, and the meaning of the pain to the patient and their family.
- Assessment of patients with chronic pain should include a history, a physical examination with particular attention to neurological function, a psychosocial assessment and, when appropriate, diagnostic testing such as imaging.

Key references

Blyth FM, March LM, Cousins MJ. Chronic pain-related disability and use of analgesia and health services in a Sydney community. *Med J Aust* 2003;179:84–7.

Breivik H, Bond MJ. Why pain control matters in a world full of killer diseases. *Pain Clinical Updates* 2004;XII:1–4.

Cepeda MS, Africano JM, Polo R et al. What decline in pain intensity is meaningful to patients with acute pain? *Pain* 2003;105:151–7.

Cousins MJ, Brennan F, Carr DB. Pain relief as a human right: a survey of medical, ethical and legal background and strategies. *Eur J Pain*. 2007; in press.

Rogers WH, Wittink HM, Ashburn MA et al. Using the "TOPS", an outcomes instrument for multidisciplinary outpatient pain treatment. *Pain Med* 2000;1:55–67.

Siddall PJ, Cousins MJ. Persistent pain as a disease entity: implications for clinical management. *Anesth Analg* 2004;99:510–20.

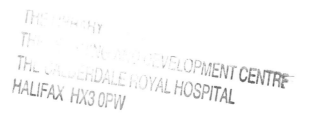

THE LIBRARY
THE ... AND DEVELOPMENT CENTRE
THE CALDERDALE ROYAL HOSPITAL
HALIFAX HX3 0PW

Trigeminal neuralgia is an idiopathic, paroxysmal recurrent pain in the distribution of one or more branches of the trigeminal (fifth cranial) nerve (Figure 3.1).

Pathophysiology

There is no firm consensus as to the mechanisms that initiate and maintain trigeminal neuralgia. Pain is thought to be caused by vascular

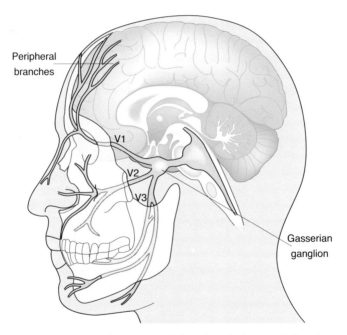

Peripheral branches

V1

V2

V3

Gasserian ganglion

Figure 3.1 Location and structure of the trigeminal nerve. It has three branches (or divisions): the upper first branch (ophthalmic; V1), which runs above the eye, forehead and front of the head; the middle second branch (maxillary; V2), which runs through the cheek, upper jaw, teeth and gums, and side of the nose; and the lower third branch (mandibular; V3), which runs through the lower jaw, teeth and gums. All three branches meet at the Gasserian ganglion.

compression of the trigeminal ganglion or its branches (Figure 3.2), but bony abnormalities or otherwise inapparent multiple sclerosis (MS) could also be contributors. Surveys of MS clinics have shown that 2% of patients with MS have trigeminal neuralgia; furthermore, in 0.2% of these patients trigeminal neuralgia was diagnosed before MS was diagnosed.

Compression of the peripheral branches of the trigeminal nerve can also occur intraorally or in the mental region alongside the chin as the result of trauma, metastatic tumor or injury during alveolar or mandibular bone excision during tooth extraction.

About 5% of people with trigeminal neuralgia have other family members with the disorder, which suggests a possible genetic cause in some cases.

Injury to the nerve root renders axons and axotomized neurons in the Gasserian ganglion hyperexcitable. A discharge from the Gasserian ganglion is then thought to spread to neighboring neurons, triggering them to fire in turn. Therefore, although trigeminal neuralgia may have an initially inapparent peripheral origin, the clinical syndrome results

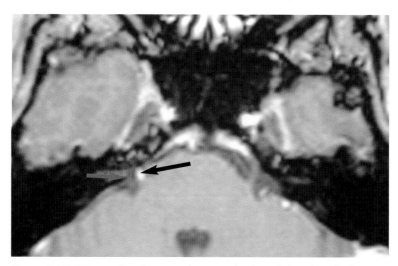

Figure 3.2 MRI scan showing vascular compression of the trigeminal ganglion in a patient with trigeminal neuralgia. The red arrow points to the right trigeminal nerve (gray area); the black arrow points to the vascular loop (branch of the posteroinferior cerebellar artery; white area).

from abnormal discharges within clusters of central neurons and/or abnormal central processing of afferent neural impulses.

Diagnosis

Because there are no objective tests for trigeminal neuralgia, clinical manifestations are the mainstay of diagnosis. Trigeminal neuralgia is more prevalent in women than men by a ratio of 3:2. It can occur at any age, but usually has its onset in individuals over 50 years old.

Clinical features. Trigeminal neuralgia is characterized by paroxysmal and recurrent attacks of facial pain that are sudden and unilateral, and that follow the distribution of one or more divisions of the trigeminal nerve. Pain is precipitated from trigger areas or by innocuous daily activities such as eating, talking, washing the face or brushing the teeth. Patients are asymptomatic between paroxysms. The pain is often severe. Patients describe it as sharp, stabbing or burning in quality, usually lasting between a few seconds and less than 2 minutes.

Differential diagnosis. If the pain is bilateral or continuous and if there are no evident provoking factors, other diagnoses should be considered, such as idiopathic facial pain, dental pain, atypical facial pain or one of the headache syndromes (e.g. cluster or migraine). If there are ocular disturbances, systemic symptoms (e.g. fever, anorexia, weight loss) and tenderness to palpation of the temporal area, temporal arteritis should be considered.

Imaging. The most important diagnostic imaging technique is magnetic resonance imaging (MRI). MRI can identify benign or malignant lesions or plaques of MS. In addition, high-resolution MRI (e.g. three-dimensional, fast-inflow MRI with steady-state precession) now enables a much more detailed study of the trigeminal nerve and its spatial relation with vascular structures (see Figure 3.2). However, the true benefits of these new techniques are uncertain because of study limitations; for example, studies in which the evaluator was already aware of gold-standard test results or in which there was an inadequate comparator.

Key points – trigeminal neuralgia

- Trigeminal neuralgia is characterized by paroxysmal and recurrent attacks of facial pain that are sudden and unilateral, and follow the distribution of one or more divisions of the trigeminal nerve.
- Pain is caused by compression of the trigeminal ganglion or its branches.
- Medical management remains the first line of treatment, with carbamazepine as the drug of choice.
- The efficacy of invasive procedures for trigeminal neuralgia has not been adequately assessed.

Pharmacological management

Medical management remains the first line of treatment, with meta-analyses of randomized controlled trials showing the anticonvulsant carbamazepine, 800–1200 mg/day, to be the drug of choice. In general, 1 of every 3 individuals receiving carbamazepine will experience pain relief. Frequent adverse events include sedation and dizziness. Rare adverse events are decreased platelet or white blood cell counts and skin problems.

Lamotrigine, slowly titrated to reach 100–400 mg/day, may offer an additional effect in patients who obtain insufficient relief with carbamazepine. Other options include the gabapentinoids (gabapentin or pregabalin), particularly in older people or in patients who are unable to tolerate carbamazepine.

Invasive procedures

Surgery is employed when medical treatment fails. However, the effectiveness of these invasive procedures has been assessed only in case series rather than in controlled clinical trials, and the optimal surgical approach has not yet been identified. A review of the literature has suggested that, of the destructive procedures, those at the level of the ganglion (radiofrequency thermocoagulation, balloon compression and neurolysis with glycerol) are more effective than those at the periphery (peripheral neurectomy, cryoanalgesia and alcohol neurolysis), but neither approach can be relied on to produce long-term pain relief.

In non-responders, or in patients for whom the pain relief is only temporary, a new or repeat procedure is sometimes performed, but the long-term efficacy of this strategy is unknown, and the risk of producing new neurological deficits is higher. Patients who elect to undergo repeat procedures should be informed of the increased risks.

Complications. All of these procedures are neurodestructive and can result in sensory loss and dysesthesia. Surgical decompression is thought to have longer-term benefits, but no head to-head comparison has been made with, for example, radiofrequency thermocoagulation.

Key references

Devor M, Amir R, Rappaport ZH. Pathophysiology of trigeminal neuralgia: the ignition hypothesis. *Clin J Pain* 2002;18:4–13.

Peters G, Nurmikko TJ. Peripheral and gasserian ganglion-level procedures for the treatment of trigeminal neuralgia. *Clin J Pain* 2002;18:28–34.

Sindrup SH, Jensen TS. Pharmacotherapy of trigeminal neuralgia. *Clin J Pain* 2002;18:22–7.

Zakrzewska JM. Diagnosis and differential diagnosis of trigeminal neuralgia. *Clin J Pain* 2002;18: 14–21.

The term 'complex regional pain syndrome' (CRPS) was coined in 1995 by the International Association for the Study of Pain to replace previous terminology used to describe the condition (Table 4.1). CRPS requires the presence of several factors.

- Regional spontaneous pain (often with a burning quality), allodynia or hyperalgesia that is disproportionate to the injury and extends beyond the territory of a single peripheral nerve.
- Evidence of edema, changes in skin blood flow or abnormal sweating in the region of the pain (Figure 4.1).
- The absence of other conditions that would otherwise account for the degree of pain and dysfunction.

A conservative estimate of the combined incidence of CRPS types I and II is 6 new cases per 100 000 people.

Pathophysiology

CRPS may be triggered by a variety of events, such as trauma, surgery, inflammatory processes, cerebrovascular accidents and nerve injury. No precipitating factor can be identified in approximately 10% of cases.

TABLE 4.1

Terminology used to describe complex regional pain syndrome

Type I
- Formerly 'reflex sympathetic dystrophy' (RSD)*
- Refers to cases with no definable nerve lesion

Type II
- Formerly 'causalgia'
- Refers to cases with a defined nerve lesion

*The term RSD, now obsolete, implied a pathophysiological mechanism (sympathetic nervous system hyperactivity) that was unverifiable, so an operational description was introduced.

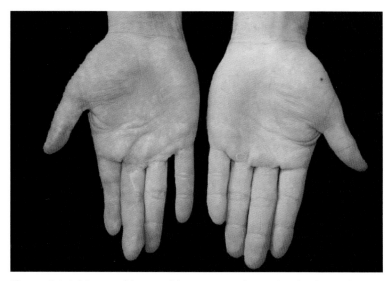

Figure 4.1 A 23-year-old man with type I complex regional pain syndrome. He had a 1-year history of pain in his right hand following direct trauma. He presented with edema and changes in temperature and skin color. The right hand is reddish, with muscle atrophy.

After initial controversy, psychological factors are no longer viewed as etiologic contributors (see 'Psychological processes' below). In addition to the pathogenic mechanisms common to all types of neuropathic pain, there are some features that are particularly characteristic of CRPS. Animal studies have shown that nerve injury is followed by:

- sprouting of noradrenergic axons around sensory neurons at the corresponding dorsal root ganglia
- upregulation of α_2-adrenoreceptors
- an abnormally intense response of injured axons to sympathetic stimulation.

The abnormal innervation and excitation by sympathetic stimulation provide a possible explanation for the abnormal discharges in peripheral nerves that are observed following nerve damage.

In humans, the nature and extent of involvement of the sympathetic nervous system is less clear. Pain alleviation after sympathetic nerve blockade or sympatholytic drug therapy is not consistent, and relapses are common. Consequently, other theories have been proposed.

Inflammatory processes. Many of the signs of CRPS resemble those of neurogenic inflammation: erythema, hyperthermia and edema. When C fibers are stimulated, the impulse propagation is bidirectional. The antidromic propagation causes the C fibers to release neuropeptides (e.g. substance P, calcitonin gene-related peptide and bradykinin), which promote vasodilation, increase capillary endothelial permeability in the skin and produce edema. Therefore, the signs and symptoms of CRPS could in part reflect an exaggerated regional inflammatory response, which manifests as a subacute inflammatory process. However, the beneficial effects of epidural clonidine and spinal cord stimulation suggest that central processes also play an important role.

Psychological processes. There is general agreement that CRPS is associated with emotional and behavioral changes, but it is not clear whether these psychological symptoms are the cause or the result of the pain syndrome. The psychological symptoms observed in patients with CRPS are also common in patients with other chronic pain syndromes, thereby supporting the idea that psychological dysfunction is the result of prolonged pain and disability and not the cause of the syndrome itself. Nevertheless, experts have called attention to the high prevalence of concurrent financial factors such as workers' compensation or injury-related litigation, and the presence of 'psychogenic pseudoneuropathy' in patients with these syndromes. This clinical entity is characterized by non-anatomic motor or sensory problems but no organic dysfunction. Signs of nerve dysfunction such as sensory loss, weakness or dystonia can be abolished by distraction.

Depending upon whether or not sympathetic blockade produces pain relief, the syndrome is described as sympathetically maintained or sympathetically independent. It is believed that sympathetically maintained pain may coexist with pain syndromes other than CRPS, such as postherpetic neuralgia.

Diagnosis

A number of diagnostic tests have been evaluated in patients with CRPS, but diagnosis of the condition remains a clinical one. Radiological abnormalities such as cortical thinning and cortical bone loss (due to increased osteoclastic activity) are often present in CRPS. Patients with CRPS have an abnormal third phase of bone scintigraphy, which is characterized by increased periarticular uptake involving multiple joints in the affected extremity. However, a critical review of bone scintigraphy in the diagnosis of CRPS reported wide variability in scintigraphic changes and very low sensitivity and specificity. Loss of function and changes in regional blood flow could explain the imaging findings.

Treatment

Despite increasing knowledge of its pathophysiological mechanisms, case series of patients with CRPS suggest that over a third fail to improve with therapy.

Physical therapy. Clinical consensus supports the benefit of mobilization and resumption of activity in the compromised limb (particularly weight- or load-bearing exercise). However, hardly any randomized controlled trials (RCTs) have evaluated the effect of physical therapy on CRPS. One RCT found that physical therapy has, at most, a short-term benefit.

Pharmacological management

Calcitonin is a hormone produced in the thyroid gland. It has a hypocalcemic effect by inhibiting osteoclastic bone resorption and increasing urinary excretion of calcium and phosphorus. Calcitonin also has a central analgesic effect, but the mechanism for this is unknown. Naturally occurring porcine calcitonin, synthetic salmon calcitonin and synthetic human calcitonin are all in clinical use. Calcitonin is usually administered by intramuscular or subcutaneous injection, but the intranasal route is also frequently used. RCTs to evaluate the benefits of calcitonin in patients with CRPS have shown a small effect at best.

Corticosteroids. Two small, single-blind RCTs reported a decrease in pain in patients with CRPS after treatment with corticosteroids. The limited sample size of these two studies (23 and 36), and the fact that the studies were not double-blind, must be taken into account when considering the significance of the results.

Key points – complex regional pain syndrome

- Reflex sympathetic dystrophy and causalgia are variants of complex regional pain syndrome (CRPS; see Table 4.1).
- The involvement of the sympathetic nervous system in CRPS is likely, but detailed mechanisms vary among patients and remain unclear.
- Diagnosis requires the presence of pain, evidence at some time of edema, changes in skin blood flow or abnormal sweating in the region of the pain, and the absence of any other condition that might account for the symptoms.
- Intravenous regional sympathetic blockade with guanethidine or systemic phentolamine lack efficacy.
- Local anesthetic blockade of the sympathetic chain is the default clinical treatment for CRPS, but the scarcity of randomized controlled trials precludes any firm conclusion regarding its effectiveness.
- Sympathectomy by surgical division, chemical neurolysis or radiofrequency lesioning should be avoided.

Bisphosphonates. CRPS is associated with increased bone resorption and patchy osteoporosis. Three double-blind RCTs reported that patients treated with alendronate intravenously (7.5 mg/day for 3 days) or orally (40 mg/day) had less pain, tenderness and swelling than those receiving placebo, and an improvement in motion; however, the very small sample sizes (20 to 32) in these studies preclude any firm conclusion that bisphosphonates are useful therapies for CRPS.

Tricyclic antidepressants. Although antidepressants are known to be effective in the treatment of neuropathic pain, only one trial has been conducted in patients with CRPS. It evaluated 48 patients with CRPS type II. Subjects who took clomipramine exhibited greater pain relief than did those who received aspirin.

Anticonvulsants. Although anticonvulsants are efficacious treatments for neuropathic pain, their use for the treatment of CRPS has not been evaluated, with the exception of one trial that evaluated gabapentin in

307 subjects with neuropathic pain, 85 of whom had CRPS types I or II. Subjects who received gabapentin exhibited greater improvement than did those who received placebo.

Capsaicin. A meta-analysis of therapies for CRPS and peripheral neuropathy demonstrated that topical application of capsaicin (an alkaloid derived from chile peppers) decreased pain intensity. However, it was difficult to conduct a blind study because of the burning sensation associated with capsaicin treatment.

Modulation of the sympathetic nervous system. The efficacy of phentolamine and of intravenous regional sympathetic block with guanethidine has not been confirmed in RCTs.

Local anesthetic blockade of the sympathetic chain is a standard clinical therapy for CRPS, but the scarcity of RCTs precludes any conclusion concerning the efficacy of this intervention. A qualitative systematic review of observational studies published on this topic has suggested that less than a third of patients treated by sympathetic blockade with local anesthetics obtain full pain relief. This rate of success is acceptable to many patients and clinicians, yet its magnitude could be attributed to placebo response, natural history or regression to the mean.

Invasive procedures. The therapies discussed below should not be considered part of the early treatment of CRPS because they are invasive, there is a scarcity of evidence to support their use and, to date, only short follow-up periods have been reported. These therapies should therefore only be offered in the context of multidisciplinary treatment and after careful screening and patient selection. Nevertheless, the dilemma associated with the use of invasive techniques is that they seem to be more successful when applied early in the course of the condition. Thus, a stepwise approach to non-invasive treatment should be pursued with deliberate speed.

Surgical sympathectomy. Definitive sympathectomy by surgical division, neurolytic nerve blocks or radiofrequency lesioning is not recommended, as none of these techniques provides long-lasting pain relief; in fact, surgical sympathectomy frequently leads to new or worsened chronic pain.

Spinal cord stimulation. Invasive treatments such as peripheral nerve stimulation with an implantable, programmable generator and spinal cord stimulation have been reported in the form of case series. Up to 15% of the systems have to be removed owing to lack of lasting pain relief. The only RCT conducted to date reported that 37% of a small sample of 36 patients achieved substantial improvement in their global assessment but no improvement in functional status.

Nevertheless, in severe and refractory cases of CRPS a trial of spinal cord stimulation may be reasonable. Objective evidence of improvement should first be documented in a temporary trial (e.g. abolition of tremor, improved range of movement, ability to bear weight) before proceeding with the implantation of stimulating electrodes.

Epidural clonidine. The same judicious approach as described for spinal cord stimulation should be taken for the use of epidural clonidine. Although some case series have reported beneficial effects, there are no rigorous data for patients with CRPS. However, a trial of epidural clonidine may be appropriate in patients with intractable CRPS.

Key references

Baron R, Levine JD, Fields HL. Causalgia and reflex sympathetic dystrophy: does the sympathetic nervous system contribute to the generation of pain? *Muscle Nerve* 1999;22:678–95.

Cepeda MS, Carr DB, Lau J. Local anesthetic sympathetic blockade for complex regional pain syndrome. *Cochrane Database Syst Rev* 2005, issue 4. CD004598.
www.thecochranelibrary.com

Cepeda MS, Lau J, Carr DB. Defining the therapeutic role of local anesthetic sympathetic blockade in complex regional pain syndrome: a narrative and systematic review. *Clin J Pain* 2002;18:216–33.

Furlan AD, Mailis A, Papagapiou M. Are we paying a high price for surgical sympathectomy? A systematic literature review of late complications. *J Pain* 2000;1: 245–57.

Kingery WS. A critical review of controlled clinical trials for peripheral neuropathic pain and complex regional pain syndromes. *Pain* 1997;73:123–39.

Ochoa JL. Pain mechanisms in neuropathy. *Curr Opin Neurol* 1994;7:407–14.

Perez RS, Kwakkel G, Zuurmond WW, de Lange JJ. Treatment of reflex sympathetic dystrophy (CRPS type 1): a research synthesis of 21 randomized clinical trials. *J Pain Symptom Manage* 2001;21:511–26.

Schott GD. An unsympathetic view of pain. *Lancet* 1995;345:634–6.

Stanton-Hicks M, Janig W, Hassenbusch S et al. Reflex sympathetic dystrophy: changing concepts and taxonomy. *Pain* 1995;63:127–33.

Veldman PH, Reynen HM, Arntz IE, Goris RJ. Signs and symptoms of reflex sympathetic dystrophy: prospective study of 829 patients. *Lancet* 1993;342:1012–16.

Verdugo RJ, Campero M, Ochoa JL. Phentolamine sympathetic block in painful polyneuropathies. II. Further questioning of the concept of 'sympathetically maintained pain'. *Neurology* 1994;44:1010–14.

Verdugo RJ, Ochoa JL. 'Sympathetically maintained pain'. I. Phentolamine block questions the concept. *Neurology* 1994;44:1003–10.

Walker SM, Cousins MJ. Complex regional pain syndromes: including "reflex sympathetic dystrophy" and "causalgia". *Anaesth Intensive Care* 1997;25:113–25.

Diabetic neuropathy

Diabetic neuropathy refers to a group of heterogeneous disorders that affect the autonomic and peripheral nervous systems of patients who have diabetes mellitus. Approximately 20% of patients with diabetes experience diabetic neuropathy, which may or may not be painful. Over 45% of individuals who have had diabetes for 25 years will experience painful diabetic neuropathy.

Patients report a spectrum of symptoms ranging from mildly disturbing tingling to severe pain that can interfere with sleep and normal activities. The degree of damage does not correlate with pain intensity, and patients can develop insensitive feet without preceding pain or paresthesias. Table 5.1 lists the major types of painful diabetic neuropathy.

Pathophysiology. Persistent hyperglycemia is the primary factor responsible for nerve damage. Hyperglycemia increases oxidative stress in nerve cells because of an excess of polyol (sugar alcohol) in the aldose reductase pathway and increased production of diacylglycerol, which subsequently activates protein kinase C.

In 11% of diabetic patients, neurological signs are evident before the diagnosis of diabetes, which suggests that the pathogenic mechanism in some patients is only loosely linked to hyperglycemia.

Glycemia-independent theories include autoimmune damage, damage due to hypoxia, and decreased synthesis of nerve growth factor and neurotrophins.

Diagnosis of diabetic neuropathy rests heavily on a careful medical history. The American Academy of Neurology recommends that patients with diabetes and neuropathy should provide a medical history and undergo a neurological examination, as well as a nerve conduction velocity study, quantitative sensory testing and quantitative autonomic

TABLE 5.1

Types of painful diabetic neuropathy

Type	Description/symptoms
Acute mononeuropathy	• Normal tendon reflexes • Vascular obstruction • Truncal neuropathy
Autonomic neuropathy	• Silent myocardial infarction • Gastroparesis • Bladder dysfunction • Disturbed neurovascular flow
Compressive neuropathy	• Sensory loss in nerve distribution (e.g. carpal tunnel syndrome)
Large fiber neuropathy	• Motor weakness • Impaired vibration perception
Small fiber neuropathy	• Paresthesias • No motor deficit • Defective heat sensation • Later, progressive hypoalgesia • Risk of foot ulceration
Proximal motor neuropathy	• Pain in thighs • Weakness • Diminished tendon reflexes • Diabetic amyotrophy

function testing. The last two tests evaluate the patient's reaction to vibration, light touch, pain and changes in temperature, as well as proprioception and autonomic function.

To allow primary care providers to detect neuropathy in diabetic subjects in clinical practice easily, a simple diagnostic tool has been developed and validated – the diabetic neuropathy symptom score. Primary care providers should ask patients about unsteadiness in walking, and the presence of pain, paresthesia or numbness. Each symptom adds one point for a maximum possible score of 4. A score of 1 or higher is considered diagnostic for polyneuropathy.

During the physical examination, clinicians can simply, rapidly and reliably screen patients for polyneuropathy using the vibration test. This test comprises the application of a 128-Hz tuning fork to the bony prominence bilaterally situated at the dorsum of the toe just proximal to the nail bed. The patient should then be asked to report the perception of both the onset and the subsiding of the sensation of vibration. Testing should be conducted twice on each toe. If more than half of the responses are incorrect (five incorrect responses or more out of ten tests), it is considered diagnostic for peripheral neuropathy.

Prevention. Complications of diabetes mellitus (including infections) are more common with poor glycemic control. Randomized controlled trials (RCTs) have shown that maintenance of near-normal blood glucose levels with intensive insulin treatment is the best approach to primary and secondary prevention of late diabetic complications such as diabetic neuropathy, the prevalence of which may be reduced by 64%.

Metabolic treatment. The use of metabolic treatments seems to be a promising approach. Aldose reductase inhibitors suppress the accumulation of alcohol sugars in nerve cells and thus improve conduction velocity; however, the clinical importance of these surrogates is inconclusive.

Pharmacological management. Tricyclic antidepressants and anticonvulsants are the medications of choice for neuropathic pain, but side effects are common.

Tricyclic antidepressants

Efficacy. The effectiveness of antidepressants for diabetic neuropathy has been confirmed in meta-analyses of RCTs. Trial findings have indicated that 1 in 4 individuals given antidepressants experiences substantial pain relief (at least 50% relief). However, 1 in 3 individuals develops minor side effects and 1 in 17 stops the medication because of the severity of side effects. The most well-studied antidepressants are amitriptyline, imipramine and desipramine. Doses of amitriptyline studied range from 25 to 150 mg/day.

Newer antidepressants such as selective serotonin-reuptake inhibitors (SSRIs) are preferable to tricyclic antidepressants for the treatment of depression, but SSRIs do not inhibit the reuptake of both serotonin and norepinephrine (noradrenaline), which appears to be necessary for efficacy against diabetic neuropathy. Emerging data on the treatment of neuropathic pain with the 'balanced' serotonin–norepinephrine-reuptake inhibitor duloxetine are promising.

Adverse effects associated with the use of antidepressants are primarily dry mouth and sedation, both of which are the result of the drugs' antimuscarinic activity. Low starting doses and careful titration may help to minimize these effects. Orthostatic hypotension and tachycardia, sometimes associated with tricyclic antidepressants, may also pose a problem in the elderly. Because disturbances of cardiac rhythm may be potentiated by tricyclic antidepressants, a baseline electrocardiogram should be taken before such therapy is started, particularly in the elderly.

Mechanism of action. The analgesic benefit of tricyclic antidepressants can be explained by several pharmacological mechanisms: they inhibit the presynaptic uptake of norepinephrine and serotonin within nociceptive monoamine pathways and thereby augment analgesia; they interact with opioid receptors; and they block calcium and sodium channels.

Anticonvulsants

Efficacy. The effectiveness of anticonvulsants has been confirmed in meta-analyses of RCTs. As with antidepressants, 1 in 3 individuals given anticonvulsants experiences pain relief. However, 1 in 4 individuals experiences minor adverse effects or severe symptoms that cause them to stop taking the medication.

A traditionally employed anticonvulsant for neuropathic pain is carbamazepine, 400–1000 mg/day. The more recently introduced anticonvulsant gabapentin, 2400–3600 mg/day, is also widely used for neuropathic pain; evidence from RCTs suggests that it is not superior to carbamazepine in terms of effectiveness or common side effects. It is not clear if pregabalin is superior to gabapentin. However, pregabalin does not require lengthy titration. Trial data show that 1 in 5 individuals given pregabalin, 150–600 mg/day, experiences pain relief.

Adverse effects. Infrequent cases of Stevens–Johnson syndrome and lymphoid hyperplasia have been reported in patients treated with carbamazepine, but not in those treated with gabapentin or pregabalin.

One in 10 individuals taking gabapentin or pregabalin stops taking the medication because of severe adverse events such as dizziness, somnolence or ataxia. The adverse events are dose related: trial data have shown that, with daily doses of 150 mg, only 1 in 39 individuals taking pregabalin discontinues the medication due to adverse events. Perhaps because the clinical picture indicates fewer severe adverse events with gabapentin and pregabalin, clinicians have widely adopted these gabanoids as first-line agents for the treatment of neuropathic pain.

Treatment of patients with neuropathic pain and cardiovascular disease should begin with anticonvulsants, given the increased risk of cardiovascular events associated with the use of tricyclic antidepressants.

Mechanism of action. Many anticonvulsants block voltage-dependent sodium channels and suppress peripherally generated ectopic impulse activity. However, some anticonvulsants such as gabapentin and pregabalin exert their effect through non-sodium-channel mechanisms. They act upon a modulatory site of neuronal calcium channels. Gabanoid binding at this site reduces calcium influx at nerve terminals and reduces the release of excitatory neurotransmitters.

Opioids

Efficacy. Opioids are increasingly used for the treatment of refractory pain regardless of etiology. The effectiveness of opioids in neuropathic pain is beginning to be evaluated in RCTs, but their long-term efficacy and side effects have not been well defined. To date, trials of opioids for neuropathic pain, which have tended to be only several weeks long, have demonstrated intermediate efficacy, with 1 in 6 individuals on opioids obtaining substantial pain relief; however, side effects are common.

A meta-analysis of RCTs has shown that tramadol, an analgesic with a dual mechanism of action (i.e. activating both opioid receptors and descending inhibitory pain systems) reduces pain intensity in patients with postherpetic neuralgia and diabetic neuropathy at mean doses of 210 mg/day. As with studies that have evaluated traditional opioids, the follow-up periods in the tramadol studies were short. No conclusion can therefore be made as to whether there is a decline in effectiveness with chronic use due to tolerance, as might be expected for that portion of the drug's effect that is opioid related.

Adverse effects. Systematic reviews of RCTs have revealed that about 80% of patients receiving opioids experience at least one adverse event. The small number of patients in these trials, and the short duration of follow-up, mean that key concerns regarding tolerance and addiction have not yet been answered.

Mechanism of action. Opioid receptors are coupled to ion channels via G proteins. When activated, these receptors modulate calcium and potassium entry into the neuron's membrane. Opioids decrease nociceptive transmission and produce analgesia by hyperpolarizing nociceptive cell membranes, shortening the duration of their action potentials and inhibiting the release of excitatory mediators. However, opioids can also induce a state of increased pain sensitivity (hyperalgesia) even after a relatively short period of exposure. Explanations for this paradoxic effect include prolongation of the neuronal action potential, activation of descending facilitatory pathways, modulation of N-methyl D-aspartate receptors and increased release of dynorphin in the spinal cord. Opioid-induced hyperalgesia may limit the long-term efficacy of these drugs in some patients with chronic pain.

Key points – diabetic neuropathy

- Persistent hyperglycemia is the primary factor responsible for nerve damage in diabetes mellitus.
- Maintenance of near-normal blood glucose levels is the best approach to primary and secondary prevention of diabetic neuropathy.
- Diabetic neuropathy affects the autonomic and peripheral nervous systems.
- Tricyclic antidepressants and anticonvulsants are the medications of choice for neuropathic pain, but side effects are common.
- The use of opioids for the treatment of neuropathic pain remains controversial because the literature has not established the long-term safety and efficacy of these drugs.

Postherpetic neuralgia

Postherpetic neuralgia is pain that persists after the vesicular rash of acute herpes zoster (shingles) has resolved. Rarely, the condition occurs despite the absence of an obvious rash. The associated pain intensity is usually mild or moderate, but may be excruciating. Typically, a single dermatome is involved, but occasionally more than one is affected.

Pathophysiology. Acute herpes zoster results from reactivation of varicella zoster virus that has remained latent in neurons of the spinal dorsal root ganglia since an earlier infection, usually childhood chickenpox (in more than 90% of cases). Risk factors for virus activation are older age, malignant disease including lymphoma, and immunosuppression due to drugs or disease.

When reactivated, the virus replicates and spreads outwards to sensory ganglia and afferent peripheral nerves. The virus causes neuronal loss and inflammatory infiltrates in the dorsal root ganglia, nerves and nerve roots. These changes trigger the pathophysiology associated with neuropathic pain (see Chapter 1, pages 14–18). Interestingly, animal studies have suggested that even in the latent phase the presence of the virus may induce abnormalities in afferent nerve function.

Natural history. Advancing age is an important risk factor for developing postherpetic neuralgia. After acute herpes zoster infection, 2% of patients under 60 years old develop postherpetic neuralgia, but this figure progressively triples with older age. The apparent requirement for postherpetic analgesia reported in RCTs is higher, perhaps reflecting a referral bias. Other risk factors are the severity of the acute zoster lesions and the intensity of the acute pain.

The duration of postherpetic neuralgia is highly variable, but 3% of all individuals with this type of pain will continue to have severe pain 1 year after the onset of herpes zoster.

Diagnosis. Postherpetic neuralgia is diagnosed on the basis of a history of shingles and the presence of persistent neuropathic pain in the affected dermatome. Symptoms are experienced around the area of skin

47

Key points – postherpetic neuralgia

- Postherpetic neuralgia is pain that persists after the vesicular rash of herpes zoster has resolved.
- During an attack of acute herpes zoster (shingles) reactivation of the varicella zoster virus, previously dormant in the dorsal root ganglia, induces inflammation and neuronal destruction.
- Tricyclic antidepressants and anticonvulsants are useful therapies.
- The efficacy of tricyclic antidepressants and anticonvulsants in postherpetic neuralgia is similar to that reported for other neuropathic pain syndromes.

---

where the shingles outbreak first occurred. Patients describe a sharp, jabbing, burning pain or a deep, aching pain, with extreme sensitivity to touch and temperature change. They sometimes describe an itching sensation or numbness, and in instances of cranial nerve involvement their complaints may be considered simply as headaches.

Pre-emptive treatment. Meta-analyses of RCTs have indicated that aciclovir, 800 mg five times daily for 7 days, during an acute herpes zoster attack reduces the risk of developing postherpetic neuralgia.

One RCT found that a 90-day course of amitriptyline begun during the acute herpes zoster attack reduces pain intensity 6 months later.

Pharmacological management

Sympathetic blockade. Anecdotal observations of prompt pain reduction and apparent truncation of the evolution of acute shingles into postherpetic neuralgia have led to the use of sympathetic blockade during the acute phase of this viral illness. However, RCTs to support this practice are lacking.

Corticosteroids. Meta-analyses of RCTs evaluating the use of systemic corticosteroid therapy for acute herpes zoster have found that corticosteroids do not prevent postherpetic neuralgia.

Tricyclic antidepressants are useful therapies for postherpetic neuralgia. Meta-analyses of RCTs have indicated similar efficacy to that reported for diabetic neuropathy (see page 43). As with diabetic neuropathy, SSRIs do not seem to be effective in postherpetic neuralgia.

Anticonvulsants. Meta-analyses of RCTs have confirmed the efficacy of anticonvulsants for relieving postherpetic pain. The efficacy for anticonvulsants in postherpetic neuralgia is similar to that reported for diabetic neuropathy (see page 44).

Capsaicin, the substance in chile peppers that makes them taste 'hot' even at room temperature, relieves pain in patients with postherpetic neuralgia. Capsaicin binds to vanilloid receptors on C and Aδ fibers, and provokes pain at initial application because of the release of substance P from the peripheral nerve terminals. This thermal cue makes blinding in RCTs difficult and may positively bias the benefits observed in such trials. Pain relief upon repeated application of capsaicin reflects depletion of excitatory mediators from peripheral nerve endings.

Opioids. Discussion on the use of opioids in diabetic neuropathy (see pages 45–6) applies equally to their use in postherpetic neuralgia or other neuropathic chronic pain.

Lidocaine skin patch. A meta-analysis of RCTs of topical lidocaine patches for postherpetic neuralgia reached no firm conclusion as to their efficacy.

Non-pharmacological management. Trials to evaluate the effectiveness of transcutaneous electrical nerve stimulation (TENS) for chronic pain have been inconclusive owing to the small number of subjects, a lack of placebo controls, a lack of long-term assessment and inadequate details of the stimulation parameters most likely to provide pain relief.

Key references

Alper BS, Lewis PR. Does treatment of acute herpes zoster prevent or shorten postherpetic neuralgia? *J Fam Pract* 2000;49:255–64.

Cepeda MS, Farrar JT. Economic evaluation of oral treatments for neuropathic pain. *J Pain* 2006;7:119–28.

Collins SL, Moore RA, McQuay HJ, Wiffen P. Antidepressants and anticonvulsants for diabetic neuropathy and postherpetic neuralgia: a quantitative systematic review. *J Pain Symptom Manage* 2000;20:449–58.

Eisenberg E, McNicol ED, Carr DB. Efficacy and safety of opioid agonists in the treatment of neuropathic pain of nonmalignant origin: systematic review and meta-analysis of randomized controlled trials. *JAMA* 2005;293:3043–52.

Greene DA, Stevens MJ, Obrosova I, Feldman EL. Glucose-induced oxidative stress and programmed cell death in diabetic neuropathy. *Eur J Pharmacol* 1999;375:217–23.

Helgason S, Petursson G, Gudmundsson S, Sigurdsson JA. Prevalence of postherpetic neuralgia after a first episode of herpes zoster: prospective study with long-term follow up. *BMJ* 2000;321:794–6.

Jung BF, Johnson RW, Griffin DR, Dworkin RH. Risk factors for postherpetic neuralgia in patients with herpes zoster. *Neurology* 2004;62:1545–51.

Kalso E, Edwards JE, Moore RA, McQuay HJ. Opioids in chronic non-cancer pain: systematic review of efficacy and safety. *Pain* 2004;112:372–80.

Santee JA. Corticosteroids for herpes zoster: what do they accomplish? *Am J Clin Dermatol* 2002;3:517–24.

Simmons Z, Feldman EL. Update on diabetic neuropathy. *Curr Opin Neurol* 2002;15:595–603.

UK Prospective Diabetes Study Group. Intensive blood-glucose control with sulphonylureas or insulin compared with conventional treatment and risk of complications in patients with type 2 diabetes (UKPDS 33). *Lancet* 1998;352:837–53.

Watson CP. The treatment of neuropathic pain: antidepressants and opioids. *Clin J Pain* 2000;16 (2 suppl):S49–55.

Wiffen P, Collins S, McQuay H et al. Anticonvulsant drugs for acute and chronic pain. *Cochrane Database Syst Rev* 2005, issue 3. CD001133. www.thecochranelibrary.com

Wood MJ, Kay R, Dworkin RH et al. Oral acyclovir therapy accelerates pain resolution in patients with herpes zoster: a meta-analysis of placebo-controlled trials. *Clin Infect Dis* 1996;22:341–7.

Zochodne DW. Diabetic neuropathies: features and mechanisms. *Brain Pathol* 1999;9:369–91.

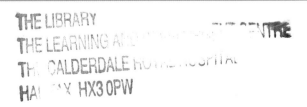
THE LIBRARY
THE LEARNING A   CENTRE
TH CALDERDALE HO   ...PITAL
HA   X HX3 0PW

Central pain results from damage to the spinal cord (Figure 6.1), or damage to the supraspinal structures, for example, as occurs after a stroke. The prevalence of central pain after traumatic spinal cord injury varies from 40–75%. Pain after spinal cord injury is of moderate-to-severe intensity in 25–60% of patients and has a deleterious effect on activities of daily living.

Pathophysiology

Preclinical and clinical studies have shown that spinal cord injury induces reorganization of the sensory and motor systems. Portions of the cerebral cortex that are normally responsive to one sensory modality often respond to other sensory modalities when deprived of their usual input. Reorganization after peripheral damage occurs either by the unmasking of connections that were previously present but functionally inactive, or by the sprouting of new connections. The unmasking of latent excitatory synapses is most likely to occur by removing the inhibition from excitatory inputs (unmasking excitation). Other possible mechanisms include increased excitatory neurotransmitter release and

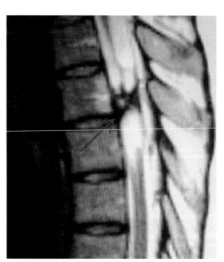

Figure 6.1 MRI scan showing spinal cord transection at the thoracic level secondary to trauma (see arrow). The patient suffered from paraplegia and spontaneous pain and allodynia in both legs.

changes in membrane conductance that enhance the effects of weak or distant inputs.

Diagnosis

Patients with central pain complain of spontaneous pain in or near the area of sensory dysfunction. The onset of pain is often not immediate, and may occur after a week or even years after the original injury; however, early onset pain that persists is also possible. The pain is often described as burning or lancinating, and worsens with light touch and movement (muscle pain, movement allodynia). In some patients, the sole manifestation is intermittent bloating in the gut, or burning urgency or fullness in the bladder.

Treatment

Very few randomized controlled trials (RCTs) have been conducted in this area, and only small numbers of patients have been enrolled. For the most part, clinicians must be guided by the evidence available from trials of drugs used to manage pain in other syndromes.

Pharmacological management

Antidepressants and anticonvulsants. A meta-analysis of RCTs has shown that tricyclic antidepressants and the anticonvulsant carbamazepine are effective for the management of central pain. The research indicates that 1 in 4 individuals treated with antidepressants or anticonvulsants will obtain substantial (at least 50%) pain relief. The same meta-analysis concluded that the selective serotonin-reuptake inhibitors mexiletine and dextromethorphan provide no benefit. Pregabalin has proved efficacious for the treatment of chronic pain after spinal cord injury; 1 in 4 individuals receiving 150–600 mg/day will obtain a 30% reduction in pain intensity.

Ketamine. Intravenous ketamine has been shown to reduce continuous and evoked pain in small crossover RCTs.

Invasive procedures

Spinal cord and deep brain stimulation. The limited evidence available from case series suggests that spinal cord stimulation has a variable rate of early success and a low rate of long-term effectiveness. Deep brain stimulation also has a low rate of early success and even lower long-term success, together with potentially serious adverse effects that include cerebrospinal fluid leak, intracranial infection, intracranial hemorrhage, persistent neurological sequelae, psychiatric complications and even death.

Dorsal root entry zone (DREZ) lesioning. The zone of dorsal root entry is the substantia gelatinosa, a column of small neurons at the most superficial extension of the dorsal gray matter that runs the length of the spinal cord.

To create DREZ lesions, a laminectomy is performed to expose the spinal cord for direct examination, and multiple lesions are made in the substantia gelatinosa by radiofrequency ablation while looking at it. It is common for lesions to be made from approximately two dermatomal levels above through to one dermatomal level below the level of spinal injury.

Impressive long-term case series have been reported, with a high percentage of patients obtaining pain relief for brachial plexus avulsion. However, clinical evaluations of DREZ lesioning have not reported the severity of adverse effects. Therefore, it is unknown whether the benefits of DREZ outweigh the risks.

Key points – central pain

- Central pain results from damage within the spinal cord or of supraspinal structures.
- 40–75% of patients with traumatic spinal cord injury develop central pain.
- Spinal cord injury is followed by reorganization of the sensory and motor systems.
- Tricyclic antidepressants and anticonvulsants, including pregabalin, are efficacious for central pain.
- Dorsal root entry zone lesioning appears to give effective pain relief after brachial plexus avulsion in case series, but its adverse effects are not well documented.

Key references

Bowsher D. Central pain: clinical and physiological characteristics. *J Neurol Neurosurg Psychiatry* 1996;61:62–9.

Chen R, Cohen LG, Hallett M. Nervous system reorganization following injury. *Neuroscience* 2002;111:761–73.

Hocking G, Cousins MJ. Ketamine in chronic pain management: an evidence-based review. *Anesth Analg* 2003;97:1730–9.

Jadad A, O'Brien MA, Wingerchuk D et al. *Management of Chronic Central Neuropathic Pain Following Traumatic Spinal Cord Injury. Evidence Report/Technology Assessment Number 45.* Maryland: Agency for Healthcare Research and Quality, 2001.

Siddall PJ, Cousins MJ, Otte A et al. Pregabalin in central neuropathic pain associated with spinal cord injury: a placebo-controlled trial. *Neurology* 2006;67:1792–800.

Siddall PJ, McClelland JM, Rutkowski SB, Cousins MJ. A longitudinal study of the prevalence and characteristics of pain in the first 5 years following spinal cord injury. *Pain* 2003;103:249–57.

Sindrup SH, Jensen TS. Efficacy of pharmacological treatments of neuropathic pain: an update and effect related to mechanism of drug action. *Pain* 1999;83:389–400.

Postincisional pain

Postincisional syndrome is defined as pain at or close to the site of a surgical incision that persists beyond the usual healing period. As with other neuropathic pain syndromes, patients exhibit allodynia and sometimes also edema in the vicinity of the surgical wound.

Pathophysiology. Trauma to nerves during the surgical procedure is thought to be the cause. The incidence of postincisional pain after surgery varies widely from 5–80%, depending upon:
- the intensity and duration of preoperative pain at the surgical site
- the effectiveness of perioperative pain control
- the location of the involved site
- genetic factors (presumed from preclinical studies).

Prevention. The results of a small randomized controlled trial (RCT) have suggested that both epidural anesthesia and epidural postoperative analgesia may have a protective effect. Subjects undergoing thoracotomy under general anesthesia plus epidural analgesia with local anesthesia, followed by postoperative epidural analgesia, were significantly less likely to develop chronic pain 6 months after the procedure than subjects who received only general anesthesia during the operation and systemic opioids postoperatively (45% versus 78%, respectively).

In addition, the use of a specific surgical approach or technique with a lower risk of nerve damage could prevent the development of chronic pain. For example, patients undergoing anterior thoracotomy are less likely to have intercostal nerve dysfunction and chronic pain than those who have a posterior/lateral thoracotomy. Similarly, deliberate preservation of the intercostobrachial nerve during breast surgery lowers the risk of developing chronic pain.

Treatment. As with other neuropathic pain syndromes, tricyclic antidepressants and anticonvulsants are first-line treatment.

Phantom pain

Phantom pain is pain in an absent body part. Up to 70% of patients develop phantom pain after limb amputation, and more than 50% of these patients experience moderate or more intense pain.

Pathophysiology. Neuromas form after amputation. These neuromas are hypersensitive and express an abnormally dense number of sodium (and other ion) channels that generate ectopic discharges. This abnormal activity initiates and maintains the central sensitization associated with nerve injury (see Chapter 1, pages 10–13). As with central pain, after amputation there is synaptic reorganization in the spinal cord, brain stem, thalamus and primary somatosensory cortex, which becomes newly responsive to neighboring body parts. These changes contribute to the persistent pain experienced after amputation.

Diagnosis. Phantom experiences, phantom pain and stump pain are different entities that share the same pathophysiological mechanisms. A phantom experience is a non-painful sensation; phantom pain is pain in an absent body part; and stump pain is local pain in the residual limb (i.e. at the amputation site). Up to 96% of amputees report phantom experiences, and 49% complain of stump pain. Depending upon the tissue amputated, phantom pain may have an early prevalence in excess of 50%. Phantom pain affects not only limbs; phantom bladder, rectal, penile, breast and vaginal pain after surgery are all well described.

While phantom sensations may be described as tingling or itchy, phantom pain consists primarily of burning, cramping and shooting pains. Phantom sensations and phantom pain typically begin within days of the amputation, and tend to decrease in frequency and duration over time, but persist for years in 40% of amputees. Sometimes phantom pain in the missing body part is similar to the pain present before the amputation.

Prevention. To date, attempts to prevent the development of phantom pain using peridural anesthesia or regional blocks have not proven successful. However, the RCTs that have evaluated these preventive measures have included a small number of subjects, and have employed regimens that have not uniformly suppressed afferent input from the involved site. Therefore, the results of the studies should be interpreted as inconclusive rather than negative.

Treatment

N-methyl D-aspartate (NMDA) receptor antagonists. Ketamine, a non-competitive NMDA antagonist, has been used in humans to treat various neuropathic pain syndromes. Intravenous ketamine provides relief from phantom and stump pain, but one small crossover RCT indicated a high incidence of side effects.

Opioids. Small randomized studies with short follow-up periods have suggested that morphine decreases pain intensity, albeit during short-term observations.

Antidepressants and anticonvulsants. There is a scarcity of controlled trial results to guide clinicians in the treatment of phantom pain, and clinicians must rely on favorable results from clinical research in which these agents have been given to treat other neuropathic pain syndromes.

Key points – traumatic nerve injury

- Postincisional pain is defined as pain at or close to the site of surgical incision that persists beyond the usual healing period; its incidence varies from 5–80%.
- Use of both epidural anesthesia and epidural postoperative analgesia may have a protective effect.
- Tricyclic antidepressants and anticonvulsants are first-line treatment.
- Phantom pain is pain in an absent body part; up to 70% of patients develop phantom pain after amputation.
- Peridural anesthesia or regional blocks before amputation have not proved successful in preventing phantom pain.
- Because of the scarcity of controlled trials in this syndrome, clinicians must rely on research on other neuropathic pain syndromes to guide pharmacotherapy of patients with phantom pain.

Key references

Dajczman E, Gordon A, Kreisman H, Wolkove N. Long-term postthoracotomy pain. *Chest* 1991;99:270–4.

Dura Navarro R, De Andres Ibanez J. [A review of clinical evidence supporting techniques to prevent chronic postoperative pain syndromes]. *Rev Esp Anestesiol Reanim* 2004;51:205–12.

Flor H, Devor M, Jensen TS. Phantom limb pain: causes and cures. In: Dostrovsky JO, Carr DB, Koltzenburg M, eds. *Proceedings of the 10th World Congress on Pain.* Seattle: IASP Press, 2003:725–38.

Fraser CM, Halligan PW, Robertson IH, Kirker SG. Characterising phantom limb phenomena in upper limb amputees. *Prosthet Orthot Int* 2001;25:235–42.

Halbert J, Crotty M, Cameron ID. Evidence for the optimal management of acute and chronic phantom pain: a systematic review. *Clin J Pain* 2002;18:84–92.

Kooijman CM, Dijkstra PU, Geertzen JH et al. Phantom pain and phantom sensations in upper limb amputees: an epidemiological study. *Pain* 2000;87:33–41.

Macrae WA. Chronic pain after surgery. *Br J Anaesth* 2001;87: 88–98.

Mehlisch DR. The combination of low dose of naloxone and morphine in patient-controlled analgesia (PCA) does not decrease opioid requirements in the postoperative period. *Pain* 2003;101:209–11.

Perkins FM, Kehlet H. Chronic pain as an outcome of surgery. A review of predictive factors. *Anesthesiology* 2000;93:1123–33.

Senturk M, Ozcan PE, Talu GK et al. The effects of three different analgesia techniques on long-term postthoracotomy pain. *Anesth Analg* 2002;94:11–15.

Cancer-related pain may arise as a direct or indirect consequence of treatment. The prevalence of cancer pain is high: 70–90% of patients with advanced cancer experience pain severe enough to interfere with several dimensions of quality of life. The severity of pain is generally lower in hematologic malignancies such as lymphomas and leukemias than in solid tumors, particularly breast or prostate cancers that commonly metastasize to bone. However, the variability of presentations of pain due to cancer and its treatment (e.g. chemotherapy-induced neuropathy or secondary infections such as herpes zoster) mandate careful, comprehensive assessment in every patient with cancer.

Pathophysiology

Metastatic spread of cancer to bone is the most common cause of cancer pain (Figure 8.1). Animal models using mice that had sarcoma

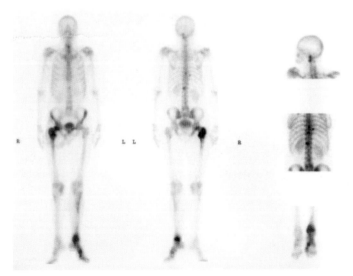

Figure 8.1 Bone scintigraphy of a 54-year-old man with prostate cancer and bone metastases. The scans show increased uptake at the sites of metastases in the cervical and lumbar spine, femur, tibia and metatarsal bone.

cells implanted into the femur showed pain behavior related both to bone destruction and to the release of inflammatory mediators derived from the tumor (e.g. prostaglandins, cytokines, endothelins). Macrophages, which are often present in large numbers in some tumor masses, also produce mediators such as tumor necrosis factor and interleukins capable of activating nociceptors.

Yet cancer pain is a nociceptive mosaic; pain may be due to tumor infiltration of nerves (neuropathic pain) or other tissues (somatic or visceral pain), or may be related to the treatment or procedure that the patient receives. Given the spectrum of potential pain sources and mechanisms, it is clear that several elements may be active in a single patient with cancer pain and that treatment should address all the pain mechanisms at play.

As with all chronic pain, psychosocial factors are of profound importance in patients with cancer pain. Saunders' concept of 'total pain' encompasses all of the factors that may affect the pain experienced by patients with cancer, including physical, psychological, social and spiritual elements.

Assessment

The same principles of pain assessment as described in Chapter 2 apply to patients with cancer pain. However, in this scenario, it is crucial to establish whether the pain is related to the cancer itself or the associated treatments. Thus, patients should be asked about the onset of pain – whether it was present before the cancer or associated with the initiation of treatments such as surgery, chemotherapy or radiotherapy – and whether it has progressed. The findings of a new physical examination may suggest a relapse or the interim development of new metastases that would warrant further investigation.

Efforts should be made to identify the specific underlying pain syndrome, as the different types may respond differently to various analgesic therapies.

In addition, open discussions with patients and their families about concerns and misconceptions surrounding the use of opioids should take place early on, as opioids are the treatment of choice for moderate-to-severe cancer pain.

Pharmacological management

Opioids are the foundation for management of cancer pain of moderate or severe intensity, especially opioids that are full agonists at the morphine receptor. Partial agonist opioids (e.g. buprenorphine) and mixed agonist–antagonist opioids (e.g. nalbuphine, butorphanol) exhibit a ceiling effect for analgesia as dose increases, although this analgesic ceiling is rarely reached at the usual clinical doses. Nalbuphine was discontinued in the UK in 2003; buprenorphine and butorphanol are available in the UK. Full opioid agonists (e.g. morphine, hydromorphone, oxycodone) do not show this ceiling effect (Figure 8.2).

Agonist–antagonist opioids also activate the κ-opioid receptor while simultaneously blocking the μ-opioid receptor, thereby risking precipitation of an opioid abstinence syndrome in patients already on a regimen of a full opioid agonist such as morphine. Therefore, only full opioid agonists at the morphine receptor should normally be used for cancer pain.

Meperidine should also be avoided in patients with cancer pain. Prolonged administration of this agent leads to accumulation of normeperidine, a toxic metabolite of meperidine with an approximate 20-hour half-life, which causes dysphoria and seizures.

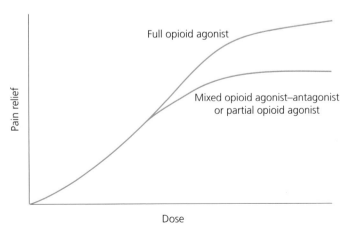

Figure 8.2 Relationship between dose and pain relief for different classes of opioid.

Mechanism of action. Opioids hyperpolarize nociceptive cell membranes, shorten the duration of their action potentials and inhibit the release of excitatory mediators. All of these actions decrease nociceptive transmission and produce analgesia.

Effect size. Study results have shown that 1 of every 3 individuals taking morphine obtains substantial pain relief.

Adverse effects. Drowsiness, nausea, vomiting, urinary retention and pruritus are frequent side effects of opioids. One of every 3 previously opioid-naive individuals develops at least one of the above side effects. The risk of respiratory depression when the opioid dose is carefully titrated to decrease cancer pain is less than 1% in the opioid-naive patient, although it is higher in older individuals (Figure 8.3). The risk of respiratory depression and all other opioid adverse effects – apart from constipation – decreases with chronic opioid administration. Constipation is almost universal during chronic opioid administration, so when chronic opioid therapy is started, a prophylactic 'bowel regimen' should also be initiated, comprising a stool softener and a stimulant cathartic.

Route of administration. Oral administration is the route of choice for chronic analgesia because of its convenience, safety, rapid onset and low cost. A systematic review of the literature has shown that the route of administration does not affect the degree of analgesia. Furthermore, controlled-release preparations are not superior to immediate-release forms in terms of pain relief or side effects, but are advantageous in terms of duration of analgesia – particularly at night.

Tolerance. Commonly, the pain-relieving effect of opioids is assumed to decline with repeated administration, that is, tolerance develops, as has been demonstrated in intact laboratory animals. Yet clinical experience indicates that tolerance to opioid analgesia is rarely the sole reason for dose escalation. The need for high doses of opioid from the start of therapy suggests an opioid-resistant pain mechanism (e.g. neuropathic pain). When abrupt dose escalation is needed, a physical reason is usually apparent (i.e. metastasis). In fact, in animal models of chronic inflammation, opioid analgesia does not decrease to any great extent during chronic exposure. Therefore, concerns about potential dose escalation and tolerance should not justify a priori

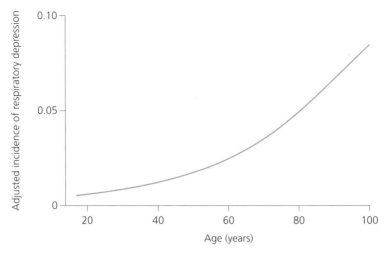

Figure 8.3 Risk of opioid (morphine)-induced respiratory depression versus age. The incidence of respiratory depression during opioid administration is low (<1%) in opioid-naive patients, but increases with age. Compared with patients aged 45 years or younger, patients between 71 and 80 years of age are 5.4 times more likely to have respiratory depression (95% confidence interval, 2.4–9.8).

decisions to withhold opioids or to restrict dose increases when they are necessary.

Opioid rotation. When the dose escalates to a level associated with unsatisfactory side effects and no physical reason is apparent, opioids should be 'rotated', that is, the dose should be tapered and the opioid discontinued while another one is started. Cross-tolerance is only partial, and rotation enables clearance of metabolites such as morphine-3-glucuronide, a morphine metabolite. If uncleared, these metabolites could antagonize opioid analgesia.

Risk of addiction. Addiction is defined as the compulsive use of a substance that results in physical, psychological and social harm to the user and continued use of the substance despite such harm. The risk of addiction in patients receiving opioids for the first time for medical purposes, such as the treatment of cancer pain, is very low.

Addiction is distinct from physical dependence, although the terms are sometimes inaccurately used interchangeably. Physical dependence is a biological phenomenon defined as the development of an abstinence syndrome following abrupt discontinuation of therapy or administration of an antagonist. Physical dependence may occur during chronic administration of many classes of drugs, including opioids, benzodiazepines, barbiturates, alcohol, β-blockers and the α_2-agonist clonidine. Physical dependence is of little clinical importance as long as abrupt discontinuation of therapy is avoided.

Breakthrough pain describes a typically brief episode of pain above a baseline pain intensity that is controlled by a long-acting or by-the-clock opioid. Treatment of breakthrough pain requires the use of rescue medication that offers a rapid onset of action and short duration. This allows patients to obtain prompt relief while avoiding lingering opioid effects once the pain intensity has returned to baseline.

Oral transmucosal fentanyl or the experimental application of intranasal ketamine seem to comply with the above requirements – both appear to offer rapid and effective relief of breakthrough pain, as shown in double-blind randomized controlled trials (RCTs).

Non-steroidal anti-inflammatory drugs

Mechanism of action. Non-steroidal anti-inflammatory drugs (NSAIDs) decrease inflammation by inhibiting the synthesis of peripheral prostaglandins. NSAIDs also have central analgesic properties that are distinguishable from their peripheral anti-inflammatory effects. They inhibit prostaglandin synthesis in the spinal cord, modulate N-methyl D-aspartate receptor activity, activate descending inhibitory pain projections and hyperpolarize cell membranes. All of these actions decrease nociceptive transmission and produce analgesia. Apart from their effects on prostaglandins, NSAIDs also affect other processes such as nuclear transcription factors and ion (K^+) channel function.

Ceiling and dose-sparing effect. NSAIDs exhibit a ceiling effect for analgesia, and therefore should not be administered above the recommended dose range. At higher doses, there is no incremental analgesic benefit and the risk of side effects increases dramatically.

Specific consensus – reached after an advisory panel was convened to address the issue of cyclooxygenase-2 (COX-2) safety – on the cardiac and cerebrovascular side effects of selective inhibitors of COX-2 has prompted withdrawal of rofecoxib and valdecoxib. Celecoxib remains on the market. Celecoxib has been associated with an increased risk of cardiovascular events in a long-term placebo-controlled trial. However, chronic use of traditional NSAIDs, with the exception of aspirin, has also been associated with an increased risk of serious cardiovascular events. Patients in need of analgesics for chronic pain should therefore be informed of the risks, and the lowest effective doses should be prescribed for the shortest appropriate duration.

NSAIDs have an opioid-sparing effect, which can be harnessed for the relief of pain of moderate or severe intensity by starting the NSAID before, or at the same time as, an opioid. The combination of an NSAID and an opioid augments pain relief by producing greater analgesia than that achieved with either drug individually. However, the results of meta-analyses question whether this benefit has been demonstrated in clinical trials.

Effect size. Meta-analyses of RCTs have shown that NSAIDs are effective for the treatment of cancer pain of mild intensity that does not originate from nerve damage. Trial findings have shown that 1 of every 3 individuals on ibuprofen and 1 of every 5 individuals on paracetamol (acetaminophen) obtain substantial pain relief.

Adverse effects. NSAID use is associated with risks of serious gastrointestinal bleeding, impaired renal function, exacerbation of hypertension or worsening of heart failure, and bleeding due to inhibition of platelet aggregation. Older patients have a particularly increased risk of serious gastrointestinal adverse effects after taking NSAIDs. Trials have shown that 1 of every 111 older patients receiving NSAIDs has serious gastrointestinal bleeding that would not have occurred otherwise.

Drugs used for treatment of neuropathic cancer pain. See pages 43–6 and 48–9 for discussion of anticonvulsants, antidepressants, cortico-steroids, capsaicin, opioids and lidocaine patches. Important 'third-line' treatments in cancer pain include low-dose ketamine infusion (150–500 µg/kg/hour) and/or lidocaine infusion (1–1.5 mg/kg/hour), either of which can be given intravenously or subcutaneously.

Bisphosphonates are analogs of pyrophosphates and are powerful inhibitors of bone resorption. Bisphosphonates are useful for the relief of pain due to bone metastases. A systematic review of the literature of RCTs, however, has shown that their effectiveness is only moderate at best, their analgesic effect is not immediate and their use is associated with frequent side effects. Therefore, they should not be considered as first-line therapy. One of every 11 individuals given bisphosphonates obtains substantial pain relief at 4 weeks and 1 of every 16 patients discontinues the therapy because of side effects.

Non-pharmacological treatment

External radiotherapy employs ionizing radiation to destroy cancer cells. A systematic review of RCTs found that radiation is efficacious to treat pain from bone metastasis. The trial data indicate that 1 of every 4 individuals treated with external radiotherapy experiences 50% pain relief within 1 month.

Radiation therapy produces pain relief by inducing apoptotic death, not only of tumor cells, thereby reducing pressure in the bone marrow, but also of highly radiosensitive inflammatory cells. However, no particular fractionation schedule has been found to be superior. The multifraction regimen is the most widely used (i.e. 30 Gy delivered in ten treatment fractions over 2 weeks).

Radionuclide therapy is the systemic use of radioisotopes; it is a form of internal radiotherapy. Radioisotopes produce pain relief with a similar degree, onset and duration as radiotherapy. However, thrombocytopenia and neutropenia are common toxic effects of radioisotopes.

A systematic review of RCTs has found that a combination of strontium radioisotopes and radiotherapy produces better quality-of-life scores than radiotherapy alone.

Hypnosis. A systematic review of the literature of RCTs has suggested that hypnosis and cognitive behavior therapy may be helpful for pain relief.

Key points – cancer pain

- Cancer pain may arise as a direct or indirect consequence of neoplasia or its treatment.
- Cancer pain is a nociceptive mosaic in which pain may arise from inflammation, tumor infiltration of nerves (neuropathic pain) or other tissues (visceral or somatic pain), treatment, or diagnostic and therapeutic procedures.
- Non-steroidal anti-inflammatory drugs exhibit a ceiling effect for analgesia and should not be administered above the recommended dose.
- Opioids are the foundation for management of cancer pain of moderate-to-severe intensity.
- Oral administration is the route of choice for chronic analgesia unless it is ineffective or contraindicated, or the patient prefers another route.
- Treatment of breakthrough pain requires the use of rescue medication with a rapid onset and short duration of action.
- Meperidine, partial opioid agonists or mixed agonist–antagonist opioids should be avoided in patients with cancer pain.
- Radiotherapy is effective in the treatment of pain from bone metastases.
- Neurolytic celiac plexus block decreases pain intensity in patients with inoperable pancreatic cancer.

Invasive procedures

Neurolytic celiac plexus block. The celiac (or solar) plexus is the largest of the great plexuses of the sympathetic nervous system. It contains afferent and efferent visceral fibers. Neurolytic celiac plexus block aims to destroy the nociceptive visceral fibers. A systematic review of the literature of RCTs and a double-blind controlled trial have shown that the procedure, which is indicated for the treatment of visceral pain of malignant origin, decreases pain intensity in patients with inoperable pancreatic cancer.

The patient is placed in a prone position and after local infiltration anesthesia just caudal to the tips of the 12th ribs, 20-gauge needles are inserted bilaterally. Under fluoroscopic guidance, the needles are advanced 1 to 2 cm anterior to the anterior margin of the L1 vertebral body, taking care not to inadvertently puncture the aorta on the left or vena cava on the right. After administering a local anesthetic test dose and observing a positive response, either in the same session or the following day, alcohol is injected for the neurolysis. Deliberate transaortic or even anterior approaches have also been employed, the latter with the aid of real-time computed tomography.

Key references

American Pain Society. *Guideline for the Management of Cancer Pain in Adults and Children*. Illinois: American Pain Society, 2006. www.ampainsoc.org/pub/cancer.htm

American Pain Society. *Principles of Analgesic Use in the Treatment of Acute Pain and Cancer Pain*. 5th edn. Illinois: American Pain Society, 2006. www.ampainsoc.org/pub/principles.htm

Carr DB, Cousins MJ. Spinal route of analgesia. Opioids and future opioids. In: Cousins MJ, Bridenbaugh PO, eds. *Neural Blockade in Clinical Anesthesia and Management of Pain*. 3rd edn. Philadelphia: Lippincott Raven, 1998:915–83.

Carr DB, Goudas LC, Balk EM et al. Evidence report on the treatment of pain in cancer patients. *J Natl Cancer Inst Monogr* 2004;(32):23–31.

Cepeda MS, Farrar JT, Baumgarten M et al. Side effects of opioids during short-term administration: effect of age, gender, and race. *Clin Pharmacol Ther* 2003;74:102–12.

Clark D. 'Total pain', disciplinary power and the body in the work of Cicely Saunders, 1958–1967. *Soc Sci Med* 1999;49:727–36.

Cleeland CS. The impact of pain on the patient with cancer. *Cancer* 1984;54(11 suppl):2635–41.

Gabriel SE, Jaakkimainen L, Bombardier C. Risk for serious gastrointestinal complications related to use of nonsteroidal anti-inflammatory drugs. A meta-analysis. *Ann Intern Med* 1991;115:787–96.

Goudas LC, Carr DB, Bloch R et al. *Management of Cancer Pain. Evidence Report/Technology Assessment Number 35*. Maryland: Agency for Healthcare Research and Quality, 2001.

Jacob AK, Carr DB, Payne R et al. *Management of Cancer Pain. Clinical Practice Guidelines.* AHCPR Publication No 94-0595. Maryland: Agency for Health Care Policy and Research, 1994.

Lawrence DP, Goudas LC, Lipman AJ et al. Management of cancer pain. In: Chang AE, Ganz PA, Hayes DF, Kinsella TJ et al., eds. *Oncology: An Evidence-Based Approach.* New York: Springer, 2005:1446–72.

McNicol E, Horowicz-Mehler N, Fisk RA et al. Management of opioid side effects in cancer-related and chronic noncancer pain: a systematic review. *J Pain* 2003;4:231–56.

McNicol E, Strassels SA, Goudas L et al. NSAIDs or paracetamol, alone or combined with opioids, for cancer pain. *Cochrane Database Syst Rev* 2005, issue 1. CD005180. www.thecochranelibrary.com

McQuay HJ, Carroll D, Moore RA. Radiotherapy for painful bone metastases: a systematic review. *Clin Oncol (R Coll Radiol)* 1997;9:150–4.

Portenoy RK, Dole V, Joseph H et al. Pain management and chemical dependency. Evolving perspectives. *JAMA* 1997;278:592–3.

Wong R, Wiffen PJ. Bisphosphonates for the relief of pain secondary to bone metastases. *Cochrane Database Syst Rev* 2002, issue 2. CD002068. www.thecochranelibrary.com

THE LIBRARY
THE LEARNING AND DEVELOPMENT CENTRE
THE CALDERDALE ROYAL HOSPITAL
HALIFAX HX3 0PW

Chronic low back pain

There are many definitions of chronic back pain depending on the context and investigators' perspective. Symptoms of pain in the lower back are more prevalent than those in the mid or upper back. Chronic back pain is defined by orthopedic surgeons as back pain that lasts longer than 7–12 weeks. Frequent recurring back pain is also classified as chronic pain since it intermittently affects an individual over a long period. Chronic back pain has also been defined as pain that lasts beyond the expected period of healing. Furthermore, insurance and industrial sources consider individuals to have chronic back pain if their symptoms result in loss of work or disability.

Given this variety of definitions, estimates of prevalence vary (Table 9.1). In contrast to the prevalence of osteoarthritis (see page 85), that of back pain decreases with age (see Table 9.1). One epidemiological study in the Netherlands found that as many as 25% of individuals with new-onset low back pain were symptomatic at 12 months, although in most cases pain resolved within 2 months.

Pathophysiology. Chronic low back pain is a complex biopsychosocial process that cannot be explained on purely anatomic, biomechanical, neurophysiological, immunologic, inflammatory or neurochemical

TABLE 9.1

Estimates of prevalence for chronic low back pain

Prevalence	Range
Point	12–33%
1-year	22–65%
Lifetime	11–84%
In people < 80 years old	14–51%
In people ≥ 80 years old	7–22%

grounds. For example, job dissatisfaction is a strong risk factor for individuals with acute back pain to develop chronic pain. Low income and poor education are also risk factors for chronic back pain and disability. For these reasons some researchers argue that chronic disability from back pain is primarily related to a psychosocial dysfunction, but the validity and reliability of this statement is uncertain.

Models of low back pain indicate that mechanical and neurochemical factors interact closely. Mechanical trauma could lead to the production of metalloproteinases and cytokines; the actions of these substances on the extracellular matrix of the intervertebral disk produce disk degeneration and pain.

When the etiology of low back pain is apparent, it is most often a musculoskeletal abnormality of the lumbar spine such as muscle strain, arthritis or disk degeneration; however, low back pain may also be referred from visceral pathology, including vascular problems such as abdominal aortic aneurysm.

Like other chronic pain syndromes, chronic back pain may also involve central neuroplastic changes such as neuronal hyperactivity, changes in membrane excitability and expression of new genes that perpetuate pain even in the absence of new tissue injury.

Diagnosis. The diagnosis of chronic back pain is a clinical one. Although anatomic abnormalities can be readily identified by imaging studies, there is no causal relationship between radiographic findings and non-specific low back pain, because most radiological abnormalities are common in asymptomatic people. Reaching a specific diagnosis is often impossible.

The diagnostic strategy recommended by the US Agency for Healthcare Policy and Research in 1994 (now the Agency for Healthcare Research and Quality) remains valid today. It is appropriate to start symptomatic therapy without imaging tests in adults under 50 years of age who lack signs or symptoms of systemic disease.

For patients over 50 years of age, or for those whose history or physical findings raise the possibility of systemic disease, plain radiography and simple laboratory tests can almost completely rule out any serious underlying conditions such as cancer.

Indications for magnetic resonance imaging (MRI) or computed tomography (CT) scanning are shown in Table 9.2. Although physicians and patients prefer MRI to radiographic evaluations, MRI scans offer little additional benefit to patients. In fact, the use of MRI may elevate the costs of care because of the increased number of spine operations that patients are likely to undergo.

If pain is not substantially improved within 6 weeks, further diagnostic evaluation is appropriate; the choice of imaging study depends on the clinical syndrome. Although MRI is a logical next step, CT scanning is less expensive and almost as accurate in identifying most underlying conditions, making it a reasonable alternative.

Preventive treatment

Exercise. A systematic review of randomized controlled trials (RCTs) has found that exercise and physical activity are of moderate utility for the prevention of chronic back pain.

Lumbar supports and back schools. There is strong evidence from RCTs that lumbar supports and back schools are not effective pre-emptive interventions. A back school is a structured educational

TABLE 9.2

Indications for imaging* in patients with back pain

- Major trauma
- Age > 50 years
- History of cancer
- Unexplained weight loss
- Fever
- Immunosuppression
- Saddle anesthesia[†]
- Bowel or bladder incontinence
- Severe or progressive neurological deficit

*Magnetic resonance imaging and computed tomography.
[†]A physical symptom of numbness in the area of the groin and upper inner thighs, consistent with the portion of the body that would come into contact with a saddle.

program, usually in a group setting, designed to inform patients about low back problems.

Smoking and weight reduction. Although smoking and excess weight are predictors of back pain, there is no persuasive evidence that modifying these risk factors relieves pain.

Non-pharmacological treatment

Exercise. As with the findings for acute back pain, in which a return to usual activity is the most effective therapy, meta-analyses of RCTs of exercise have shown that exercise programs reduce pain and improve function in patients with subacute, chronic or persistent postsurgical low back pain.

Supervised stretching and strengthening fitness programs achieve the largest improvement compared with unsupervised exercise. One RCT has found that lumbar flexion in the early morning (i.e. a form of self-care) reduces pain intensity and costs associated with chronic non-specific low back pain.

Massage and spinal manipulation. A meta-analysis of trials that evaluated massage has concluded that the technique is beneficial for subacute and chronic back pain. Methodological flaws of the included trials (lack of randomization or blinding) weaken the findings. Systematic reviews and a large RCT of 1334 participants have concluded that spinal manipulation produces a small-to-moderate benefit at 3 months; however, its efficacy decreases over time and at 12 months the benefit is only small.

A separate meta-analysis concluded that spinal manipulation does not reduce neck pain; moreover, case reports have documented rare but serious cerebrovascular events due to arterial damage induced by cervical manipulation.

Acupuncture. A recent meta-analysis has indicated that acupuncture produces both short-term (6 weeks) and long-term (6 months) relief of chronic back pain even when sham acupuncture is used as a comparator. However, the available data are insufficient to compare the efficacy of acupuncture with pharmacotherapy or non-drug therapies.

Cognitive behavior therapy. A meta-analysis of RCTs has indicated that cognitive therapy reduces both pain intensity and behavioral expression of pain in patients with chronic pain (including those with back pain).

Other treatments. According to systematic reviews of the literature, transcutaneous electrical nerve stimulation (TENS) and the use of special corsets both lack effectiveness for the management of chronic back pain.

Pharmacological management

Non-steroidal anti-inflammatory drugs (NSAIDs). Although NSAIDs are effective for short-term symptomatic relief of acute low back pain, a systematic review of RCTs of NSAIDs for chronic back pain found insufficient evidence to support their use for this purpose.

RCTs that evaluate the combination of paracetamol (acetaminophen) plus weak opioids such as codeine or tramadol have found that these combinations reduce pain intensity. However, long-term effectiveness is unknown because of the short duration of the studies and the likelihood that tolerance would diminish the apparent analgesic benefit of such combinations during long-term clinical use.

Antidepressants. A systematic review of RCTs suggests that while antidepressants reduce the severity of chronic back pain, they do not improve functional status.

Invasive treatment

Epidural steroid injections. One out of 8 patients who receive epidural steroid injections will experience at least 75% of pain relief in the short term, but this benefit fades over time as only 1 out of 13 patients will obtain 50% of pain relief in the long-term (12 weeks to 1 year).

Spinal cord stimulation is increasingly used for the treatment of chronic back pain, especially in patients with failed back pain syndrome (persistent pain and functional limitation after spinal surgery). A small RCT reported that patients with spinal cord stimulation are less likely to undergo reoperation. However, the value of this outcome is difficult to interpret since function and employment status were similar in both groups (patients randomized to reoperation or spinal stimulation).

Surgical treatment. Prospective cohort studies and RCTs have shown that for patients with moderate-to-severe sciatica, surgical treatment yields greater improvement than non-surgical treatment. On the other hand, conservative therapies should be considered the first line of treatment, as selecting a conservative treatment does not run the risk of surgical complications and the relative short-term benefit of surgery decreases over time.

There is no evidence that spinal fusion, one of the most common operations for low back problems, is superior to other surgical procedures such as laminectomy for common degenerative conditions of the spine. Interestingly, the outcome of spinal stenosis surgery does not seem to be associated with the degree of postsurgical spinal canal narrowing.

Future treatment. Recently an 'artificial disk' has been approved for marketing, with the goal of preserving relatively normal spine architecture and mechanics after operations involving shrunken or extruded disks. Use of gene therapy such as adenovirus-mediated gene transfer to nucleus pulposus cells to halt or slow disk degeneration is also an attractive prospect.

Spinal stenosis

Spinal stenosis refers to congenital (rare) or acquired (common with advanced age) narrowing of the spinal canal or the foramina through which the nerve roots exit (Figure 9.1).

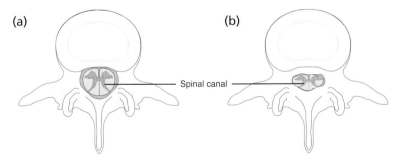

Figure 9.1 Cross-section of a vertebra with (a) a normal spinal canal and (b) stenosis of the canal and associated nerve compression.

Five of every 1000 people over 50 years of age are estimated to have symptoms of spinal stenosis.

Pathophysiology. Typically, the condition occurs in the cervical or lumbar spine as a result of invasion of the spinal canal by osteophytes, tissue from hypertrophied facets, bulging disks and/or hypertrophy of the ligamentum flavum, the ligament that connects the laminae of the vertebrae and prevents excessive motion between the vertebral bodies. Compression of the medullary and lumbar cord or nerve roots produces symptoms of chronic neck or back pain along with cervical or lumbar radiculopathy, respectively.

Diagnosis. Patients with spinal stenosis experience numbness, weakness of the extremities and (for lumbar stenosis) leg pain upon walking. The latter symptom, termed 'neurogenic' claudication, occurs because, when the patient walks erect, increased epidural, intrathecal and foraminal pressures compromise microcirculation to the spinal cord and nerve roots. Patients with leg pain upon walking as a result of inadequate blood flow to one or both legs are said to have 'vascular' claudication.

Symptoms of lumbar stenosis typically occur upon standing or walking downstairs, and improve when the patient leans forward (e.g. on a shopping cart in a supermarket). Leaning forward (or simply sitting down) tends to create more space in the spinal canal and foramina, thereby decreasing compression of neural tissue and the local blood supply that feeds it.

Treatment of spinal stenosis follows the same principles as described above for back pain with the exception of one type of spinal stenosis termed 'cauda equina syndrome', which requires immediate surgical decompression. The cauda equina is so named because of the resemblance of the nerve roots at the caudal end of the spinal cord, which float freely within spinal fluid, to the tail of a horse.

Cauda equina syndrome is seen when severe pressure on the nerve fibers at the base of the spinal column results in loss of control of the bowel or bladder, pain, severe weakness, or loss of feeling in one or both legs. This is a medical emergency, and surgery – or radiation therapy and high-dose glucocorticoids when the cause is inoperable cancer – is indicated to relieve the pressure and prevent irreversible loss of spinal cord function.

Key points – chronic low back pain* and spinal stenosis

- When the etiology of low back pain is apparent, it is most often a musculoskeletal abnormality of the lumbar spine; however, low back pain may also be referred from visceral pathology.
- Chronic low back pain is a complex biopsychosocial process that cannot be explained on purely anatomic, biomechanical, neurophysiological, immunologic, inflammatory or neurochemical grounds.
- Symptomatic therapy can be initiated without imaging tests in adults under 50 years of age who lack signs or symptoms of systemic disease.
- For patients over 50 years of age, or whose findings suggest systemic disease, plain radiography and simple laboratory tests can almost completely rule out underlying systemic disease.
- CT or MRI should be reserved for patients over 50 years of age, or those with major trauma, a history of cancer, unexplained weight loss, fever, immunosuppression, saddle anesthesia, bowel or bladder incontinence or a severe progressive neurological deficit.
- Exercise has moderate utility in the prevention or treatment of chronic back pain.
- Massage, spinal manipulation and acupuncture provide small-to-moderate short-term benefits.
- There is insufficient evidence to support the use of non-steroidal anti-inflammatory drugs for the treatment of chronic low back pain.
- Epidural steroid injections produce small-to-moderate short-term pain relief.
- Antidepressants reduce pain severity but do not improve function.

*See *Fast Facts: Low Back Pain* for further information.

Fibromyalgia

Fibromyalgia is characterized by:

- chronic widespread pain
- multiple tender points
- fatigue
- poor-quality sleep.

The condition is more common in women, and its incidence appears to increase through middle age, after which it declines. The prevalence of fibromyalgia in the general population ranges from 0.5–5%, but it could be as high as 10% in women between 55 and 64 years of age. Symptoms may last for years, and relapses are common.

There is debate as to whether fibromyalgia constitutes a unique clinical entity or disease process because of the considerable overlap between patients with fibromyalgia and those with other unexplained syndromes such as irritable bowel syndrome, chronic fatigue syndrome and atypical chest pain.

Pathophysiology. The pathophysiology of fibromyalgia remains uncertain. To date, the multidimensional (mechanical, thermal and electrical) hyperalgesia observed in patients with fibromyalgia has been explained in terms of a diffuse central sensitization leading to centrally generated symptoms and/or abnormal processing of normal sensory input. Brain imaging studies support this explanation. Altered cytokine profiles may underlie peripheral or central sensitization.

The fatigue and sleep disturbances associated with this condition have been attributed to alterations in the hypothalamic–pituitary–adrenal (HPA) axis caused by hyperactivity of neurons that express corticotropin-releasing hormone. Cytokines have the capacity to disrupt the normal function of the HPA axis.

Diagnosis. Fibromyalgia is a clinical syndrome with no known laboratory test to confirm the diagnosis. Clinical diagnosis is made on the basis of a history of widespread pain and pain triggered by digital palpation of at least 11 of 18 tender points (Figure 9.2). The pain tends to be diffuse, aching or burning, and is often described as 'head to toe'. The pain intensity can vary, and can change location on the body.

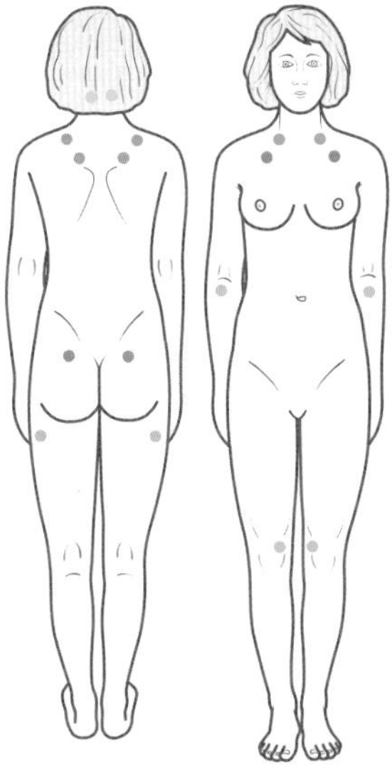

- Occiput:
  suboccipital muscle
- Trapezius:
  midpoint of the upper
  border
- Supraspinatus:
  above the medial border
  of the scapular spine
- Gluteal:
  upper outer quadrants
  of buttocks
- Greater trochanter:
  posterior to trochanteric
  prominence

- Low cervical:
  anterior aspects of
  the intertransverse
  spaces at C5–C7
- Second rib:
  second costochondral
  junctions
- Lateral epicondyle:
  2 cm distal to
  epicondyles
- Knee:
  medial fat pad
  proximal to the
  joint line

Figure 9.2 Tender points that indicate the presence of fibromyalgia.

Pharmacological management

Non-steroidal anti-inflammatory drugs. Paracetamol and NSAIDs are commonly used to relieve pain in patients with fibromyalgia. However, RCTs have found no clear benefit of NSAIDs over placebo for this condition. When combined with antidepressant agents, NSAIDs may confer a slight incremental analgesic benefit. However, some authors argue that the marginal additional benefit of NSAIDs in the long term, given their potential toxicity, is not cost-effective.

Tricyclic antidepressants. A meta-analysis of RCTs has confirmed that antidepressants relieve stiffness, reduce tenderness and improve sleep quality in fibromyalgia. On the other hand, evidence for the effectiveness of selective serotonin-reuptake inhibitors is conflicting.

Weak opioids. RCTs evaluating the efficacy of tramadol and paracetamol have found that the combination of these two drugs is superior to placebo in decreasing pain intensity. However, the follow-up period was short, and the potential for tolerance and dependence has not yet been elucidated (see pages 61–4 for a more detailed discussion of these issues).

Anticonvulsants. The gabapentinoid pregabalin has been shown to produce small-to-modest benefits in patients with fibromyalgia. The results of an RCT have suggested that pregabalin reduces pain, improves sleep and reduces fatigue in patients with fibromyalgia. One of every 6 individuals given pregabalin obtains pain relief, but minor adverse events also occur with the same prevalence.

Non-pharmacological treatment

Exercise. RCTs have demonstrated that aerobic exercise improves physical symptoms and anxiety scores. However, the minimal or optimal exercise regimen to produce such benefits has not yet been defined.

Acupuncture. There is conflicting evidence on the efficacy of acupuncture for fibromyalgia. A systematic review of the literature could not account for the wide diversity of study results.

Education may include strategies for coping with symptoms, encouraging physical activity and discussion of biomedical knowledge with health providers. However, a systematic review of the efficacy of these types of program produced disappointing results since their benefits were not maintained at follow-up.

Prognosis. With appropriate treatment, mild-to-moderate fibromyalgia is not necessarily physically debilitating. The condition does not reduce life span.

Key points – fibromyalgia

- Fibromyalgia is characterized by chronic widespread pain, tender points, fatigue and poor quality of sleep.
- There is debate as to whether fibromyalgia constitutes a unique disease process.
- Fibromyalgia is a clinical syndrome; there is no laboratory test that confirms the diagnosis.
- Exercise and tricyclic antidepressants are effective treatments.

Pain due to osteoporosis

Osteoporosis is a systemic skeletal condition characterized by decreased bone density and weakened bone structure that leads to an increased risk of bone fracture.

The most common primary forms of bone loss are postmenopausal and age-related osteoporosis. Osteoporosis may also be secondary to a wide variety of medical problems, including hypercortisolism, hyperthyroidism, hyperparathyroidism, alcohol abuse and immobilization.

Approximately 25% of postmenopausal women have osteoporosis, and in people 60 years of age or older it is the most common risk factor for non-traumatic fractures. Osteoporosis produces chronic pain due to fractures. Vertebral fracture is the most frequent complication of osteoporosis (Figure 9.3). Population studies have demonstrated that vertebral fractures are associated with high rates of chronic pain, functional decline, psychosocial dysfunction and early mortality.

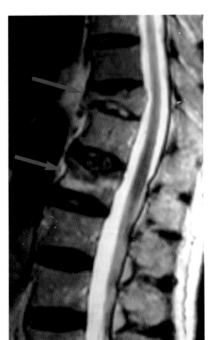

Figure 9.3 MRI scan showing two osteoporotic vertebral fractures in the thoracic region (red arrows). The lower fracture is a recent one.

Diagnosis. The earliest symptom of osteoporosis is often an episode of acute, severe back pain caused by a vertebral compression fracture, or acute, severe groin or thigh pain caused by a hip fracture. Diagnostic work-up should include a clinical history, physical examination, laboratory evaluation, bone densitometry and radiographic imaging. This work-up will generally allow the clinician to determine the cause of osteoporosis and to institute medical interventions to slow progression or even reverse the condition.

General management. The choice of pain treatment should be tailored to the individual, as there is wide variation in the clinical presentation and the degree of physical disability associated with osteoporosis. For patients with acute or chronic pain, the treatment of pain and functional limitations should be the first priority.

Subsequent measures should include treatments aimed at maintaining bone mass to avoid new fractures, lifestyle re-education, physical therapy, physical fitness training, an appropriate course of rehabilitation to rebuild muscle mass and function, neurological and orthopedic evaluation, and, for some patients, use of an orthosis.

Pharmacological management

Non-steroidal anti-inflammatory drugs are first-line treatment for mild-to-moderate pain secondary to a stable fracture. No trials have assessed the effect of NSAIDs on the healing of osteoporotic fractures. However, retrospective cohort studies have suggested that high doses of traditional NSAIDs could increase the likelihood of non-union after spinal fusion surgery. Conversely, RCTs that have evaluated bone healing after spinal fusion have provided no evidence that cyclooxygenase-2 (COX-2) inhibitors affect the rate of non-union at 1 year.

If pain persists, an opioid should be added. For any but the briefest of courses, opioid therapy should be approached as it is for any subacute-to-chronic illness. In this mostly elderly population, the approach to opioid therapy should include the initiation of a bowel regimen at the onset of therapy (see page 62), consideration of breakthrough medication as needed and controlled-release dosage.

When prescribing NSAIDs or opioids, the usual cautions with respect to comorbidity (e.g. with renal or pulmonary disease, respectively) should be kept in mind.

Calcitonin is a natural hormone that exerts antiresorptive properties by blocking osteoclastic activity. The value of calcitonin treatment for postmenopausal osteoporosis remains uncertain, especially in the prevention of fractures. However, RCTs that have evaluated calcitonin administered after fractures indicate that, given subcutaneously or intranasally, it acts as an analgesic. Pain relief occurs within a week of starting calcitonin. Patients also seem to have earlier mobilization than those receiving a placebo.

The mechanism of action is not yet known. It could be mediated through a calcitonin effect on nociceptive transmission, or on calcitonin-binding sites in areas of the brain. Further research is required to compare the efficacy of calcitonin with standard analgesics, as 1 of every 11 individuals given calcitonin stops taking it because of adverse events such as flushing, nausea and vomiting.

Epidural analgesia. In severe, acute pain refractory to systemic medications, a short-term catheter may aid mobilization in patients who would otherwise be bed-bound. The catheter tip is usually placed as close as possible to the fracture, and small doses of an opioid and local anesthetic are infused. Evidence for the efficacy of this approach is only available from case reports.

Corticosteroid injection. Similar empirical results have shown that a single epidural injection of a corticosteroid provides symptomatic relief of inflammation adjoining a new vertebral fracture. Repeated injections, however, may enhance osteoporosis and so are relatively contraindicated.

Non-pharmacological treatment

Vertebroplasty has recently been introduced for treatment of patients with osteoporosis who have acute or chronic pain following vertebral fracture. The procedure involves the injection of bone cement into the fractured vertebral body in an attempt to stabilize fractured segments and reduce pain.

Vertebroplasty has not been evaluated in RCTs. Case series have suggested that the procedure is associated with substantial short-term pain relief and improvements in health-related quality of life (HRQoL) that seem to persist at 6 months. Other benefits include prevention of recurrent pain, reversal of height loss and spinal deformity, and improved level of function.

In general, 1–10% of patients experience short-term complications, mainly from the extravasation of cement. These problems include increased pain and damage from pressure on the spinal cord or nerve roots, infection, bleeding and pneumothorax.

Possible long-term complications include local acceleration of bone resorption caused by the treatment itself or by a foreign-body reaction at the cement–bone interface, and increased risk of fracture in treated or adjacent vertebrae through changes in mechanical forces.

Kyphoplasty (sometimes referred to as balloon-assisted vertebroplasty) has been evaluated only in case series. Before injecting the cement-like material, a balloon is inserted and gently inflated inside the fractured vertebrae. Substantial pain relief has been reported for short follow-up periods.

Kyphoplasty offers a theoretical advantage over vertebroplasty as the former is believed to provide better restoration of height and better reduction of spine deformity; however, it is more expensive. To date, no head-to-head trials have compared kyphoplasty with vertebroplasty.

Key points – pain due to osteoporosis*

- Osteoporosis increases the risk of bone fracture, of which vertebral fracture is most common.
- Non-steroidal anti-inflammatory drugs are the treatment of choice for mild-to-moderate pain secondary to a fracture, followed by opioid therapy for more severe pain.
- In case series, vertebroplasty is associated with substantial short-term pain relief and improvements in health-related quality of life that seem to persist at 6 months.

*See *Fast Facts: Osteoporosis,* 5th edition, for further information.

Pain due to osteoarthritis

Osteoarthritis is a disease characterized by joint pain, distortion of joint architecture and impaired function due to articular cartilage degeneration and local inflammation. It is the most common form of arthritis and the most common cause of disability in older adults.

Osteoarthritis affects an estimated 20 million people or more in the USA and 4.5 million people in the UK. The condition is more prevalent with advancing age: people over 35 years of age have an 11% prevalence of hip osteoarthritis that increases to 36% in people over 85 years of age. Similarly, 10% of individuals over 55 years old have knee pain due to osteoarthritis; 25% of these individuals are severely disabled.

Osteoarthritis is one of the ten leading causes of disease burden in the developed world. Pain and physical limitations produced by osteoarthritis substantially affect HRQoL. Individuals with osteoarthritis have a lower HRQoL than subjects with gastrointestinal or cardiovascular conditions, or with chronic respiratory diseases.

Pathophysiology. Although the causes of osteoarthritis are not completely understood, the enzymatic and mechanical breakdown of the cartilage matrix is key to the pathophysiology of the condition. Healthy cartilage is able to transmit force between the joints while maintaining almost friction-free limb movement. In osteoarthritis, these biomechanical properties are compromised; however, it is not clear whether the degeneration of cartilage precedes the onset of the disease or is a result of it.

The integrity of normal articular cartilage is maintained by a balance between anabolic and catabolic processes. This balance is disrupted in osteoarthritis. Cartilage degeneration correlates with age: senescent chondrocytes have decreased mitotic activity and are less responsive to anabolic growth factors, and thus synthesize smaller amounts of functional proteins. All of these changes lead to progressive cartilage damage and decreased capacity for regeneration.

In osteoarthritis, chondrocytes also produce an excess of nitric oxide and other inflammatory mediators such as eicosanoids and cytokines. The excessive nitric oxide produces cellular injury, inhibits cartilage synthesis and renders the chondrocyte susceptible to cytokine-induced apoptosis. In addition to promoting cartilage damage, these inflammatory phenomena predispose the patient to peripheral nerve sensitization with subsequent central sensitization and chronic pain.

Bone is also structurally abnormal in osteoarthritis. Periarticular bone has increased turnover, decreased bone mineral content and a reduced number of trabeculae, which affect its biomechanical integrity.

Diagnosis. Patients with osteoarthritis typically have morning stiffness and swelling of the involved joint (Figure 9.4), with pain that tends to worsen on weightbearing or activity, but improves with rest.

Physical examination often reveals tenderness on palpation, bony enlargement, crepitus with movement and/or limitation of joint motion. Unlike in rheumatoid arthritis and other inflammatory arthritides, the inflammation in osteoarthritis, if obvious at all, is usually mild and localized to the affected joint.

General management. The goals of treatment for osteoarthritis are:
- pain relief
- prevention of complications such as muscle atrophy or deformities
- maintenance and/or improvement of functional status and HRQoL.

Treatment strategies consist of pharmacological and non-pharmacological modalities and invasive procedures.

Pharmacological management

Non-steroidal anti-inflammatory drugs. Meta-analyses have shown that NSAIDs are efficacious for pain relief in osteoarthritis: 59–82% of patients receiving NSAIDs report at least 50% pain relief. Paracetamol is less effective: only 20–40% of patients who receive paracetamol report pain relief of 50% or more.

Conventional NSAIDs inhibit both of the COX isoforms COX-1 and COX-2, but COX-2 inhibitors are much more selective against the COX-2 isoform. The COX-1 isoform is expressed in a constitutive manner (i.e. always active), and is present mainly in the gastric mucosa, kidney and platelets. The COX-2 isoform is mainly expressed in an

(a)

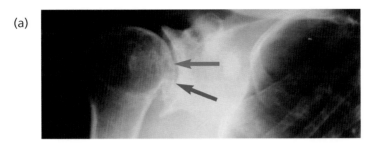

(b)

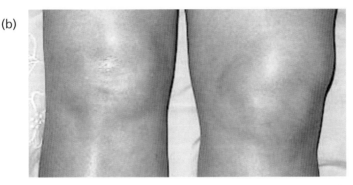

Figure 9.4 (a) Radiograph of a 65-year-old man with osteoarthritis of the shoulder. There is a marked decrease in the glenohumeral joint space (blue arrow), along with bony sclerosis (red arrow). (b) Osteoarthritis of both knees in a 67-year-old woman, with deformities and mild edema in the left knee.

inducible manner and is responsible for the enhanced formation of prostaglandins during inflammation.

Multiple RCTs have confirmed the efficacy of COX-2 inhibitors in osteoarthritis. The major clinical interest of these selective COX-2 inhibitors has been the lower incidence of gastrointestinal bleeding than that associated with traditional NSAIDs; however, this benefit is not always present, decreases over time and falls with the concomitant use of aspirin (for cardiovascular protection).

A comprehensive study of the cost-effectiveness of COX-2 inhibitors and traditional NSAIDs has found that money saved from the risk reduction of gastrointestinal adverse effects associated with COX-2 inhibitors does not offset the higher costs of these drugs during management of average-risk patients with chronic arthritis.

In addition, growing concerns regarding an increase in cardio-vascular events in patients receiving COX-2 inhibitors have led to the withdrawal of rofecoxib and valdecoxib from the market in the USA and re-evaluation of their status in Europe. On the other hand, following a thorough review in the USA and Australia, celecoxib remains on the market because of its favorable gastrointestinal safety profile.

While the efficacy and safety of NSAIDs and COX-2 inhibitors for long-term use are being re-evaluated, it seems most prudent to employ long-established NSAIDs for pain relief after careful patient selection and with ongoing monitoring. Patients receiving long-term treatment with either NSAIDs or COX-2 inhibitors should be informed that all drugs in these classes (except for aspirin) carry cardiovascular risks with chronic use.

Combination therapy. The combination of NSAIDs and weak opioids (e.g. paracetamol with codeine or tramadol) seems to provide slightly greater analgesia than paracetamol alone in patients with osteoarthritis, as double-blind RCTs have shown.

Strong opioids. Given alone or in combination with NSAIDs or paracetamol, strong opioids are efficacious for chronic arthritis pain. Controlled-release preparations (oral or transdermal) are suitable for chronic use of strong opioids such as morphine, oxycodone and fentanyl, as well as for the partial opioid agonist buprenorphine.

Glucosamine is a widely used therapy, but its efficacy is unproven.

Tricyclic antidepressants. Meta-analyses of RCTs have confirmed that tricyclic antidepressants are effective for the treatment of osteoarthritic pain.

Capsaicin. A systematic review of published RCTs found that capsaicin decreased osteoarthritic pain (see page 49 for a general description of capsaicin).

Intraarticular therapy. When patients do not respond to a program of non-pharmacological therapy (see below) and analgesics, intraarticular injections of sodium hyaluronate or corticosteroids produce symptomatic benefit that may last for as long as 6 months. However, limited data are available on the effectiveness of multiple courses of intraarticular therapy.

Key points – pain due to osteoarthritis*

- Osteoarthritis is characterized by joint pain with loss of joint architecture and function due to articular cartilage degeneration and local inflammation.
- Pain and limitation of physical function substantially affect health-related quality of life (HRQoL).
- The goal of treatment is to relieve pain, prevent complications and maintain and/or improve functional status and HRQoL.
- Exercise and weight loss are beneficial.
- Non-steroidal anti-inflammatory drugs (NSAIDs) are effective treatments for pain relief.
- Ongoing concerns regarding the safety and cost-effectiveness of chronic therapy with cyclooxygenase (COX)-2 inhibitors has led to worldwide caution concerning their use.
- Patients given long-term treatment with either NSAIDs or COX-2 inhibitors should be informed that all drugs in these classes (except for aspirin) carry cardiovascular risks with chronic use.
- Total joint arthroplasties are effective in improving HRQoL.

*See *Fast Facts: Osteoarthritis and Gout* for further information.

Surgery. Total joint replacement, such as total hip and total knee arthroplasties, are extremely effective in improving dimensions of HRQoL. Logic and evidence indicate that the timing of surgery should be individualized on the basis of response to less invasive options and with orthopedic specialist consultation.

Indications for joint replacement include radiographic evidence of joint damage and/or moderate-to-severe persistent pain or disability that are not substantially relieved by an extended course of non-surgical management.

Non-pharmacological treatment

Exercise and weight loss. Exercise reduces pain and disability in patients with osteoarthritis of the hip or knee. These findings are supported by systematic reviews of the literature and a meta-analysis of RCTs on the effect of exercise on osteoarthritic pain.

Overweight patients with hip or knee osteoarthritis who lose weight have consistently shown improvement of symptoms and function in multiple RCTs.

Education. A systematic review of published RCTs and non-randomized trials has suggested a beneficial effect of educational programs such as relaxation training, biofeedback, problem-solving strategies, social support or stress reduction for patients with osteoarthritis. These programs have been shown to reduce joint pain and the frequency of arthritis-related physician visits, increase physical activity and improve quality of life.

Acupuncture. The role of acupuncture for the treatment of osteo-arthritis is not clear. RCTs have shown that acupuncture is not superior to sham-needling in reducing osteoarthritic pain. This equivalence implies that sham-needling has similar specific effects as acupuncture or that both methods produce substantial non-specific effects.

Future treatment. In the future, efforts to prevent the development or progression of osteoarthritis will likely include strategies that delay the onset of chondrocyte senescence or replace senescent cells. These objectives can be met by disease-modifying drugs aimed at inhibiting the breakdown of cartilage or at stimulating repair activity by chondrocytes.

Pain due to rheumatoid arthritis

Rheumatoid arthritis is a chronic, systemic, autoimmune disorder characterized by joint pain and inflammation that may progress to joint destruction. Rheumatoid arthritis is the most common inflammatory arthritis and a major cause of disability; 1–2% of the world's population is affected by the condition.

Pathophysiology. A multistage theory that integrates various genetic hypotheses has been postulated. Some believe that the origin of rheumatoid arthritis is a bacterial or viral infection. Bacterial and viral antigenic particles have been detected in synovial tissue, and could be responsible for the initial activation of inflammation. B-cell activation and generation of autoantibodies directed to the Fc portion of human immunoglobulin G class molecules ('rheumatoid factors') could also be responsible for activation of innate immunity. The production of cytokines such as tumor necrosis factor-α and interleukin-1 by macrophages and fibroblasts in the joint, and the local expression of adhesion molecules following immune activation, promote the ingress of immune cells and the accumulation of T cells and B cells in the inflamed synovium. Cytokines and locally expressed degradative enzymes such as metalloproteinases digest the cartilage matrix and destroy articular and bone structures, resulting in pain.

Diagnosis of rheumatoid arthritis requires the presence of four or more of the criteria shown in Table 9.3. Subluxation of the atlantoaxial or cricoarytenoid joints may not be apparent, but patients with cervical spine instability are at risk of impingement of the spinal cord during routine procedures such as endotracheal intubation, and should therefore undergo neurological evaluation before any surgical intervention. Hoarseness or pain on talking should alert the clinician to possible problems with the cricoarytenoid joint.

TABLE 9.3

Criteria for diagnosis of rheumatoid arthritis

≥ 4 of the following features must be present:

- Morning stiffness in and around joints for ≥ 1 hour before maximal improvement*
- Soft tissue swelling of ≥ 3 joint areas*
- Swelling of the proximal interphalangeal, metacarpophalangeal or wrist joints*
- Symmetric swelling*
- Subcutaneous rheumatoid nodules
- Circulating rheumatoid factor
- Radiographic erosions and/or periarticular osteopenia in hand and/or wrist joints (Figure 9.5).

*Must have been present for at least 6 weeks.

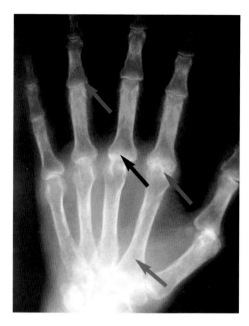

Figure 9.5 Radiograph of the hand of a 48-year-old woman with rheumatoid arthritis, showing diffuse osteopenia (red arrow), decreased interphalangeal joint spaces without sclerosis (black arrow) and subchondral cysts (blue arrows). Similar changes are observed in the carpal joints.

Pharmacological management

Non-steroidal anti-inflammatory drugs. Traditionally, pharmacotherapy for rheumatoid arthritis follows a 'pyramid model' in which the first level of treatment is NSAID therapy. Meta-analysis of RCTs has confirmed that NSAIDs are effective in decreasing pain and the number of tender joints, and improving function in rheumatoid arthritis.

COX-2 inhibitors and traditional NSAIDs have similar analgesic efficacy. However, COX-2 inhibitors should not be considered as first-line treatment (see pages 87–8 for the arguments to support this statement).

NSAID–opioid combinations. The combination of NSAIDs and weak opioids is commonly used to produce greater analgesia than can be achieved by each individual drug.

Slow-acting antirheumatic drugs (SAARDs) are used to replace or supplement NSAIDs when the latter do not provide adequate pain control. SAARDs are distinguished from NSAIDs primarily by their assumed disease-modifying potential and delayed onset of action. Agents falling within this therapeutic class include hydroxychloroquine, gold, D-penicillamine, methotrexate, azathioprine and sulfasalazine. In much of the literature this class is also termed disease-modifying antirheumatic drugs (DMARDs).

Systematic reviews of RCTs that have evaluated SAARDs have confirmed their efficacy in reducing pain intensity and decreasing the number of painful and swollen joints. However, their use is associated with a high discontinuation rate due to adverse events, especially for azathioprine and cyclophosphamide.

Oral corticosteroids decrease joint tenderness and pain, and improve grip strength with efficacy nearly equivalent to second-line agents previously examined in meta-analyses. The morbidity associated with chronic corticosteroid use mandates great caution in their use.

One RCT has suggested that SAARDs produce their greatest benefit when introduced early in the course of the disease.

Biological response modifiers (BRMs) are a third line of treatment based on pathogenic mechanisms. BRMs are DMARD treatments aimed at blocking the specific biological effects of inflammatory cytokines, tumor necrosis factor and other modulators of inflammation.

RCTs have indicated that BRMs are more efficacious than traditional agents because in addition to addressing symptoms, they attenuate synovial inflammation, halt the progression of joint damage and joint destruction, and reduce disease activity in patients with long-standing rheumatoid arthritis. One of every 4 individuals treated with BRMs will obtain substantial pain relief. However, their side effects may be serious, and include severe infection, increased risk of tuberculosis, lymphomas and demyelinating disease.

Tricyclic antidepressants. RCTs have consistently shown that antidepressants are efficacious for pain associated with rheumatoid arthritis and therefore should be an early part of the treatment armamentarium.

Non-pharmacological treatment

Education. A systematic review of the literature has concluded that patient education is efficacious in reducing pain and improving function in rheumatoid arthritis. The programs included relaxation training, biofeedback, problem-solving strategies, social support and stress reduction. Comparing its relative effectiveness with modalities such as NSAIDs, the benefit of education is 20–30% greater overall; education is also 40% greater than NSAIDs at improving functional ability and 60–80% greater at reducing tender joint counts.

A systematic review of the literature on RCTs that have evaluated the effect of relaxation, biofeedback and cognitive behavior therapies suggests that each of these therapies is an efficacious adjunctive therapy.

Occupational therapy improves functional ability in patients with rheumatoid arthritis, according to the results of a systematic review of RCTs.

Exercise. A meta-analysis of RCTs has shown that exercise in patients with well-controlled disease increases aerobic capacity, joint mobility and muscle strength.

Acupuncture has not been found to be of use for the treatment of pain associated with rheumatoid arthritis.

Key points – pain due to rheumatoid arthritis*

- Rheumatoid arthritis is a chronic, systemic, autoimmune disorder characterized by joint inflammation, joint destruction and pain.
- Education, occupational therapy, exercise, relaxation, biofeedback and cognitive behavior therapies are efficacious interventions.
- Pharmacological treatment follows a pyramidal model: it begins with non-steroidal anti-inflammatory drugs, is followed by slow-acting antirheumatic drugs and ends with biological response modifiers.
- Joint replacement is appropriate for restoration of function in joints deformed by advanced rheumatoid arthritis, but intubation for anesthesia must be approached cautiously in light of potential unappreciated cricoarytenoid or atlantoaxial joint subluxation.

*See *Fast Facts: Rheumatoid Arthritis* for further information.

Key references

American College of Rheumatology (ACR). Recommendations for the medical management of osteoarthritis of the hip and knee: 2000 update. ACR Subcommittee on Osteoarthritis Guidelines. *Arthritis Rheum* 2000;43:1905–15.

Anon. NSAIDs for treating osteoarthritis. Bandolier, 2003. www.jr2.ox.ac.uk/bandolier/booth/painpag/Chronrev/OARA/OANSAID.html

Atlas SJ, Keller RB, Chang Y et al. Surgical and nonsurgical management of sciatica secondary to a lumbar disc herniation: five-year outcomes from the Maine Lumbar Spine Study. *Spine* 2001;26:1179–87.

Cepeda MS, Camargo F, Zea C, Valencia L. Tramadol for osteoarthritis. *Cochrane Database Syst Rev* 2006, issue 3. CD005522. www.thecochranelibrary.com

Deyo RA. Diagnostic evaluation of LBP: reaching a specific diagnosis is often impossible. *Arch Intern Med* 2002;162:1444–7.

Firestein GS. Evolving concepts of rheumatoid arthritis. *Nature* 2003;423:356–61.

Fishbain D. Evidence-based data on pain relief with antidepressants. *Ann Med* 2000;32:305–16.

Hayden JA, van Tulder MW, Tomlinson G. Systematic review: strategies for using exercise therapy to improve outcomes in chronic low back pain. *Ann Intern Med* 2005; 142:776–85.

Jarvik JG, Hollingworth W, Martin B et al. Rapid magnetic resonance imaging vs radiographs for patients with low back pain: a randomized controlled trial. *JAMA* 2003;289: 2810–18.

Jenkins JK, Seligman PJ. *Analysis and Recommendations for Agency Action Regarding Non-Steroidal Anti-Inflammatory Drugs and Cardiovascular Risk.* www.fda.gov/cder/drug/infopage/COX2/NSAIDdecisionMemo.pdf

Linton SJ, van Tulder MW. Preventive interventions for back and neck pain problems: what is the evidence? *Spine* 2001;26:778–87.

Louie SG, Park B, Yoon H. Biological response modifiers in the management of rheumatoid arthritis. *Am J Health Syst Pharm* 2003;60:346–55.

Manheimer E, White A, Berman B et al. Meta-analysis: acupuncture for low back pain. *Ann Intern Med* 2005;142:651–63.

Martin JA, Buckwalter JA. Aging, articular cartilage chondrocyte senescence and osteoarthritis. *Biogerontology* 2002;3:257–64.

Messier SP, Loeser RF, Miller GD et al. Exercise and dietary weight loss in overweight and obese older adults with knee osteoarthritis: the Arthritis, Diet, and Activity Promotion Trial. *Arthritis Rheum* 2004;50:1501–10.

Molloy AR, Nicholas MK, Cousins MJ. Role of opioids in chronic non-cancer pain. *Med J Aust* 1997;167:9–10.

Salerno SM, Browning R, Jackson JL. The effect of antidepressant treatment on chronic back pain: a meta-analysis. *Arch Intern Med* 2002;162:19–24.

Spiegel BM, Targownik L, Dulai GS, Gralnek IM. The cost-effectiveness of cyclooxygenase-2 selective inhibitors in the management of chronic arthritis. *Ann Intern Med* 2003;138:795–806.

Towheed TE, Maxwell L, Anastassiades TP et al. Glucosamine therapy for treating osteoarthritis. *Cochrane Database Syst Rev* 2005, issue 2. CD002946. www.thecochranelibrary.com

Walker BF. The prevalence of low back pain: a systematic review of the literature from 1966 to 1998. *J Spinal Disord* 2000;13:205–17.

White KP, Harth M. Classification, epidemiology, and natural history of fibromyalgia. *Curr Pain Headache Rep* 2001;5:320–9.

In the past, viscera were considered insensitive to pain. It is now clear that visceral pain results from the activation of sensory afferent nerves that innervate internal organs such as the stomach, kidney, gallbladder, urinary bladder, intestines or pancreas. Disorders that could trigger visceral pain include distension from impaction, tumors, ischemia, inflammation and traction on the mesentery. There are a variety of pain syndromes thought to be maintained by the persistent activation of visceral nociceptive fibers. However, there is a common pathophysiology and symptomatic management approach to all of these syndromes.

Pathophysiology

Nociceptive input from the body surface travels along somatic nerves that enter spinal roots, accounting for the clear dermatomal organization of somatic pain sensations. Nociceptive information from internal organs, which are exclusively innervated by Aδ and unmyelinated C fibers, travels via more diffusely organized sympathetic and parasympathetic afferent pathways that enter the spine at thoracic and lumbar levels. In addition, visceral afferent fibers contain a greater percentage of neuroexcitatory transmitters such as substance P than do somatic afferent fibers. These differences between somatic and visceral innervation explain why sensations arising from visceral stimulation are generally more diffuse, more difficult to localize and more unpleasant than somatic sensations, and also why they are referred to poorly localized regions of the body surface. Visceral sensations are often accompanied by autonomic reflexes and symptoms such as nausea, sweating and malaise.

Three physiological classes of nociceptive viscerosensory receptors exist:
- high-threshold receptors that respond only to noxious mechanical stimuli
- wide dynamic range receptors that encode a wide range of innocuous and noxious stimuli
- silent receptors that are activated by inflammation.

High-threshold receptors exclusively innervate organs from which pain is the only conscious sensation (e.g. ureter, kidney, lungs, heart), but there are relatively few of this receptor type in organs that provide both innocuous and noxious sensations (e.g. colon, stomach, bladder).

The etiology of persistent visceral pain is still not certain. However, it is clear that visceral pain is not always linked to injury. It is believed that persistent activation of visceral fibers leads to central sensitization and to visceral hyperalgesia and that, just as for hyperalgesia from chronic somatic pain, excessive activity of N-methyl D-aspartate (NMDA) receptors is involved in this process. Autoimmune responses and inflammation could trigger the persistent activation of visceral afferent fibers. The possibility that visceral nerve injury may give rise to persistent visceral neuropathic pain is embodied in the term 'complex regional pain syndrome' (see Chapter 4, page 33).

Symptomatic management

Treatment of visceral chronic pain syndromes is aimed at symptomatic pain management. Today, visceral pain management focuses on both pharmacological and interventional techniques. Combinations of non-steroidal anti-inflammatory drugs, adjuvant medications and opioids, in that sequence, form the mainstay of therapy. When pharmacological therapies prove ineffective or are limited by side effects, regional anesthesia techniques, neurostimulation (peripheral or spinal cord) or neurosurgical techniques are considered. However, the efficacy of these latter therapies has not been evaluated rigorously, and therefore they should only be used as a last resort.

In addition, there are specific treatment modalities that are used for the treatment of specific pain syndromes.

For illustrative purposes, this chapter discusses the following conditions:
- irritable bowel syndrome (IBS)
- interstitial cystitis
- male chronic pelvic pain syndrome
- endometriosis.

Irritable bowel syndrome

As much as 20% of the adult population exhibits symptoms of IBS. This functional disorder is characterized by abdominal pain, cramping, bloating, constipation and diarrhea. It occurs more often in women than in men, and it begins before the age of 35 in half of those afflicted. Most people can control their symptoms with diet, stress management and medications, but for some it can be disabling, preventing them from working, attending social events or traveling even short distances.

Diagnosis. Because the condition has no pathognomonic physical signs, the diagnosis of IBS usually requires exclusion of structural pathology, which requires imaging or more invasive testing, and cannot be accomplished solely via the patient's medical history. Inclusion criteria for diagnosis are shown in Table 10.1.

Treatment. Mild symptoms of IBS usually respond to stress management and changes in diet and lifestyle. If symptoms persist

---

TABLE 10.1

Criteria for the diagnosis of irritable bowel syndrome*

- Abdominal pain[†]
- Diarrhea or constipation lasting at least 12 weeks[†]

Plus ≥ 2 of the following:
- Change in the frequency of bowel movements
- Change in the consistency of stool
- Straining
- Urgency
- A feeling of incomplete bowel movement or bloating
- Mucus in the stool

*See Fast Facts: Irritable Bowel Syndrome for more information.
[†]Do not have to occur consecutively.

despite judicious use of laxatives for constipation, antidiarrheals or antispasmodics, tricyclic antidepressants may relieve pain and diarrhea, as one of their side effects is constipation.

As the autonomic nervous system and its enteric compartment play an important role in regulating motility and visceral perception, neurotransmitters (particularly serotonin) are targets for novel pharmacotherapeutic agents for this syndrome. Specific medications for IBS include tegaserod, a partially selective serotonin agonist (not available in the UK).

Interstitial cystitis

Interstitial cystitis is a heterogeneous chronic pain syndrome that most commonly (90%) affects women. Symptoms include pain on bladder filling, pelvic pain and urinary urgency and frequency. The symptoms are often exacerbated by ovulation and during periods of stress.

Diagnosis. In the absence of practical clinical criteria for the diagnosis of interstitial cystitis, the US National Institute of Diabetes and Digestive and Kidney Diseases of the National Institutes of Health developed criteria for research purposes. These criteria were never meant to be a gold standard for diagnosis, but they are often used as such. To be diagnosed with interstitial cystitis for research purposes, patients must have glomerulations or Hunner's ulcer on cystoscopic examination, and either bladder pain or urinary urgency in the absence of other diseases that could cause the symptoms.

Treatment. Hydrodistention of the bladder, intravesical instillation therapy and transurethral resection of diseased bladder tissue have been used to treat interstitial cystitis. However, the efficacy of these therapies has not been evaluated rigorously.

Male chronic pelvic pain syndrome

The diagnosis of male chronic pelvic pain syndrome is made in men who complain of chronic pelvic pain but who have an unrevealing examination and work-up. Interstitial cystitis (see above) and male chronic pelvic pain syndrome may be the same syndrome.

Endometriosis

Endometriosis is a common gynecological condition that produces cyclic pain. Women complain of severe dysmenorrhea, focal pelvic tenderness and dyspareunia. The pain arises because of the dissemination of endometrium to ectopic sites during retrograde menstruation or surgery, and the subsequent establishment of deposits of ectopic endometrial tissue.

In many women, endometriosis is a self-limiting disease; however, in others the biological behavior is much more unpredictable.

Diagnosis is made by laparoscopy (Figure 10.1).

Treatment of endometriosis includes therapies such as medroxyprogesterone acetate, danazol, nafarelin and gonadotropin-releasing hormone analogs. Medical therapy after surgical treatment reduces pain substantially, but trials have shown that there is no difference postoperatively at 6 months whether or not medical therapy is used. Although the efficacy of a variety of treatments has been demonstrated in randomized controlled trials, only 40–70% of women with severe cases of endometriosis become pain free.

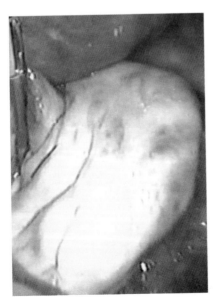

Figure 10.1 Endometriosis found on a laparoscopy of a young woman with a 6-month history of pelvic pain. The dark spots seen in the right upper quadrant of the ovary correspond to the foci of endometriosis.

Key points – visceral pain

- Visceral pain results from activation of sensory afferent nerves that innervate the stomach, kidney, gallbladder, urinary bladder, intestines or pancreas.
- Sensations arising from visceral stimulation are generally more diffuse, more difficult to localize and more unpleasant than those associated with somatic pain.
- Visceral pain is more likely than somatic pain to be associated with autonomic signs such as pallor and sweating, or symptoms such as nausea.
- Pain syndromes such as male chronic pelvic pain syndrome, interstitial cystitis, endometriosis and irritable bowel syndrome are thought to be maintained by the persistent activation of visceral fibers.

Key references

Al-Chaer ED, Traub RJ. Biological basis of visceral pain: recent developments. *Pain* 2002;96:221–5.

Batstone GR, Doble A. Chronic prostatitis. *Curr Opin Urol* 2003; 13:23–9.

Giamberardino MA. Visceral pain. *Pain: Clinical Updates* 2005;XIII: 1–6.

Howard FM. An evidence-based medicine approach to the treatment of endometriosis-associated chronic pelvic pain: placebo-controlled studies. *J Am Assoc Gynecol Laparosc* 2000;7:477–88.

Kream RM, Carr DB. Interstitial cystitis: a complex visceral pain syndrome. *Pain Forum* 1999;8: 139–45.

Peeker R, Fall M. Treatment guidelines for classic and non-ulcer interstitial cystitis. *Int Urogynecol J Pelvic Floor Dysfunct* 2000;11:23–32.

Prentice A, Deary AJ, Goldbeck-Wood S et al. Gonadotrophin-releasing hormone analogues for pain associated with endometriosis. *Cochrane Database Syst Rev* 2000, issue 2. CD000346. www.thecochranelibrary.com

Strigo IA, Bushnell MC, Boivin M, Duncan GH. Psychophysical analysis of visceral and cutaneous pain in human subjects. *Pain* 2002;97:235–46.

Wesselmann U, Czakanski PP. Pelvic pain: a chronic visceral pain syndrome. *Curr Pain Headache Rep* 2001;5:13–19.

The International Association for the Study of Pain, the American Academy of Pain Medicine, the Faculty of Pain Medicine of the Australian and New Zealand College of Anesthetists and the American College of Rheumatology, among many other professional organizations, have long advocated the multidisciplinary approach as the preferred method of restoring health-related quality of life and functionality to patients with chronic pain, since it is a multisystem condition.

The multidisciplinary team

The multidisciplinary approach to the treatment of chronic pain consists of assessing and treating the physical, psychosocial, medical, vocational and social aspects of chronic pain. The specific disciplines of healthcare providers required to offer a multidisciplinary approach are a function of the variety of patients seen and the available resources. The team may include physicians, nurses, psychologists, physical therapists, occupational therapists, vocational counselors, social workers, pharmacists and any other healthcare professional who can contribute to diagnosis or treatment. It is crucial that the members of the treatment team communicate with each other on a regular basis, both about specific patients and about overall program development.

Research evidence to support the efficacy of this approach to chronic pain treatment is just emerging. However, researchers consistently stress the need to improve the number and the quality of the trials to evaluate the effectiveness of chronic pain treatment programs.

Varied response for different syndromes

Systematic reviews of the literature suggest that the benefits of a multidisciplinary therapy are not uniform across all chronic pain syndromes. For example, for patients with chronic low back pain, behavioral treatment such as positive reinforcement of healthy behaviors, modification of patients' understanding of their pain and disability, and biofeedback, all decrease pain intensity and improve functional status. Yet, in patients with chronic neck or shoulder pain or fibromyalgia, a similar approach lacks effectiveness.

The magnitude of the effect of a multidisciplinary approach ranges from slight to moderate. The benefits are less clear when a multidisciplinary approach supplements other standard treatment. For example, behavioral treatment for chronic low back pain has a moderate effect on pain intensity, functional status and behavioral outcomes compared with being on a waiting list or simply receiving no treatment. However, when added to a usual pharmacotherapy program for chronic low back pain the positive effect is not observed.

The intensity of the multidisciplinary program also seems relevant. For example, systematic reviews of trials that evaluate multidisciplinary therapy for chronic low back pain suggest that although intensive, multidisciplinary, biopsychosocial rehabilitation with a functional restoration approach reduces pain and improves function, less intensive interventions do not produce improvement in any clinically relevant outcome.

Further research

Because of the methodological shortcomings of published trials, the cost of multidisciplinary therapy and the increasing need to prove that the cost of proposed treatments is offset by the value they add, there is an obvious need for more research to demonstrate the benefits of this approach for the treatment of chronic pain.

Key points – the multidisciplinary approach

- Since chronic pain is a multidimensional condition, expert consensus recommends the multidisciplinary approach as the method of choice to restore quality of life and functionality.
- The specific disciplines of healthcare providers required to offer a multidisciplinary approach depend on the variety of patients seen and the available resources.
- Research evidence to support the efficacy of the multidisciplinary approach to chronic pain treatment is not yet conclusive; there is an obvious need for more research to prove its cost-effectiveness.

Key references

Deyo RA. Back pain patient outcomes assessment team (BOAT). www.ahcpr.gov/clinic/medtep/backpain.htm

Guzman J, Esmail R, Karjalainen K et al. Multidisciplinary bio-psychosocial rehabilitation for chronic low back pain. *Cochrane Database Syst Rev* 2002, issue 1. CD000963. www.thecochranelibrary.com

Karjalainen K, Malmivaara A, van Tulder M et al. Multidisciplinary biopsychosocial rehabilitation for neck and shoulder pain among working age adults. *Cochrane Database Syst Rev* 2003, issue 2. CD002194. www.thecochranelibrary.com

Karjalainen K, Malmivaara A, van Tulder M et al. Multidisciplinary biopsychosocial rehabilitation for subacute low back pain among working age adults. *Cochrane Database Syst Rev* 2003, issue 2. CD002193. www.thecochranelibrary.com

Karjalainen K, Malmivaara A, van Tulder M et al. Biopsychosocial rehabilitation for upper limb repetitive strain injuries in working age adults. *Cochrane Database Syst Rev* 2000, issue 3. CD002269. www.thecochranelibrary.com

Karjalainen K, Malmivaara A, van Tulder M et al. Multidisciplinary rehabilitation for fibromyalgia and musculoskeletal pain in working age adults. *Cochrane Database Syst Rev* 2000, issue 2. CD001984. www.thecochranelibrary.com

Ostelo RW, van Tulder MW, Vlaeyen JW et al. Behavioural treatment for chronic low-back pain. *Cochrane Database Syst Rev* 2005, issue 1. CD002014. www.thecochranelibrary.com

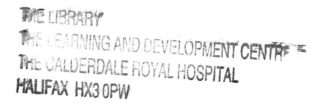
THE LIBRARY
THE LEARNING AND DEVELOPMENT CENTRE
THE CALDERDALE ROYAL HOSPITAL
HALIFAX HX3 0PW

Novel analgesics

The increased understanding of nociceptive transmission and pain pathophysiology, the recognition of heterogeneity among C fibers extending to their expression of different molecular transducers, and the discovery of new receptors such as those for vanilloids or growth factors and identification of new receptor subtypes have already resulted in preclinical and early clinical testing of novel analgesics. These agents will more specifically target receptor subtypes or ion channels, and promise to be more effective and better tolerated than present therapies. On the other hand, other novel molecules are designed to interact with multiple receptors simultaneously.

Improved technology

Advances in delivery. Setbacks that have followed the introduction of novel agents such as cyclooxygenase (COX)-2 inhibitors have been offset by the development of innovative methods to improve formulations of established compounds.

Iontophoretic or inhalational technology now permits the delivery of lipophilic opioids into the systemic circulation through the skin or lungs. Likewise, intranasal delivery of novel agents (or established agents coadministered with novel excipients) permits more rapid control of breakthrough pain than oral or transbuccal drug delivery.

Advances in imaging technology have taken us beyond a static detailed image of the central nervous system: we can now see the brain at work. Functional magnetic resonance imaging allows real-time clinical observation of the brain's pain excitatory and inhibitory circuitry, which in turn helps us to understand how nociceptive input is processed and translated into pain and suffering. Functional imaging has advanced our knowledge of placebo and analgesic responses, and has even been applied as a novel form of biofeedback to allow patients to control their otherwise refractory chronic pain.

Magnetic resonance spectroscopy appears poised to achieve the 'Holy Grail' of pain assessment: sensitive, specific diagnosis of the presence of chronic pain using a quick, simple laboratory test.

Pharmacogenetics. No doubt we will be using pharmacogenetics to prescribe analgesics in the future. Each medication will be tailored to the needs and characteristics of the individual, so that each patient will get the most benefit with the fewest side effects. Moreover, pharmacogenetics is already helping us to understand the biological basis for individual variability in response to established agents such as opioids.

Future hope

Individuals with chronic pain can look to the future with hope. Medical science has progressed from marginalizing chronic pain as merely a symptom of disease, and belittling those who seek help, to developing a better understanding of its causes and effects. Policy makers, including the World Health Organization, have come to realize the devastating effect that chronic pain has on individuals and their families, on society as a whole, and on the economy in terms of lost output and productivity.

Governments are accepting the importance of developing specialized strategies for the prevention, treatment and management of chronic pain as a fundamental human right. In addition, health services around the world are responding to calls to improve the management of painful long-term conditions; to develop preventive and cost-effective solutions; to respond to patient choice and voice; and to create healthier workplaces.

These advances should help individuals with chronic pain to overcome some of the problems they face in everyday life so that they can enjoy more opportunities, greater independence and an improved quality of life.

Key references

Bonney IM, Foran SE, Marchand JE et al. Spinal antinociceptive effects of AA501, a novel chimeric peptide with opioid receptor agonist and tachykinin receptor antagonist moieties. *Eur J Pharmacol* 2004;488:91–9.

Breivik H, Bond M. Why pain control matters in a world full of killer diseases. *Pain: Clinical Updates* 2004;XII:1–4.

Carr DB, Loeser JD, Morris DB. *Narrative, Pain, and Suffering.* Seattle: IASP Press, 2005.

Cousins MJ, Brennan F, Carr DB. Pain relief: a universal human right. *Pain* 2004;112:1–4.

Gordon DB, Dahl JL, Miaskowski C et al. American Pain Society recommendations for improving the quality of acute and cancer pain management: American Pain Society Quality of Care Task Force. *Arch Intern Med* 2005;165:1574–80.

Julius D. The molecular biology of thermosensation. In: Dostrovsky JO, Carr DB, Koltzenburg M, eds. *Proceedings of the 10th World Congress on Pain.* Seattle: IASP Press, 2003: 63–70.

Kim H, Dionne RA. Genetics, pain, and analgesia. *Pain: Clinical Updates* 2005;XIII:1–4.

Sheckler MT, Carr DB, Mermelstein FH, Hamilton DA. Nasal delivery: a boon for analgesics. *Drug Deliv* 2006;6:56–8.

Siddall PJ, Cousins MJ. Persistent pain as a disease entity: implications for clinical management. *Anesth Analg* 2004;99:510–20.

Siddall PJ, Stanwell P, Woodhouse A et al. Magnetic resonance spectroscopy detects biochemical changes in the brain associated with chronic low back pain: a preliminary report. *Anesth Analg* 2006;102:1164–8.

Stamer UM, Stuber F. Pharmacogenetics of anesthetic and analgesic agents: CYP2D6 genetic variations. *Anesthesiology* 2005;103:1099.

Villanueva L, Dickenson A, Ollat H. *The Pain System in Normal and Pathological States: A Primer for Clinicians.* Seattle: IASP Press, 2004.

Useful resources

Further reading

Carr DB, Goudas LC. Acute pain. *Lancet* 1999;353:2051–8.

Hernandez N, Vanegas H. Encoding of noxious stimulus intensity by putative pain modulating neurons in the rostral ventromedial medulla and by simultaneously recorded nociceptive neurons in the spinal dorsal horn of rats. *Pain* 2001;91:307–15.

Portenoy RK. Opioid therapy for chronic nonmalignant pain: a review of the critical issues. *J Pain Symptom Manage* 1996;11:203–17.

Tortorici V, Vanegas H. Opioid tolerance induced by metamizol (dipyrone) microinjections into the periaqueductal grey of rats. *Eur J Neurosci* 2000; 12:4074–80.

Vasquez E, Vanegas H. The antinociceptive effect of PAG-microinjected dipyrone in rats is mediated by endogenous opioids of the rostral ventromedial medulla. *Brain Res* 2000;854:249–52.

Yamamoto T, Nozaki-Taguchi N. Analysis of the roles of cyclooxygenase (COX)-1 and COX-2 in spinal nociceptive transmission. In: Jensen TS, Turner JA, Wiesenfeld-Hallin Z, eds. *Proceedings of the 8th World Congress on Pain*. Seattle: IASP Press, 1996: 303–12.

Useful addresses

UK

The British Pain Society
Third Floor, Churchill House
35 Red Lion Square
London WC1R 4SG
info@britishpainsociety.org
www.britishpainsociety.org

Chronic Pain Policy Coalition
Ground Floor, Irwin House
118 Southwark Street
London SE1 0SN
Tel: +44 (0)20 7202 9412
info@paincoalition.org.uk
www.paincoalition.org.uk

Pain Concern
PO Box 13256
Haddington EH41 4YD
Tel: +44 (0)1620 822572 (Mon–Fri 9 AM–5 PM, Fri 6.30–7.30 PM)
info@painconcern.org.uk
www.painconcern.org.uk

The Pain Relief Foundation
Clinical Sciences Centre
University Hospital Aintree
Lower Lane, Liverpool L9 7AL
Tel: +44 (0)151 529 5820
secretary@painrelieffoundation.org.uk
www.painrelieffoundation.org.uk

USA

Agency for Healthcare Research and Quality
540 Gaither Road, Suite 2000
Rockville, MD 20850
Tel: +1 301 427 1364
www.ahrq.gov

American Academy of Orofacial Pain
19 Mantua Road
Mount Royal, NJ 08061
Tel: +1 856 423 3629
aaopco@talley.com
www.aaop.org

American Academy of Pain Medicine
4700 W Lake Avenue
Glenview, IL 60025
Tel: +1 847 375 4731
info@painmed.org
www.painmed.org

American Alliance of Cancer Pain Initiatives
Room 4720, 1300 University Avenue
Madison, WI 53706
Tel: +1 608 265 4013
aacpi@mailplus.wisc.edu
www.aacpi.wisc.edu

American Chronic Pain Association
PO Box 850, Rocklin, CA 95677
Toll-free: 1 800 533 3231
ACPA@pacbell.net
www.theacpa.org

American Pain Foundation
201 North Charles Street, Suite 710
Baltimore, MD 21201-4111
Toll-free: 1 888 615 7246
info@painfoundation.org
www.painfoundation.org

American Pain Society
4700 W Lake Avenue
Glenview, IL 60025
Tel: +1 847 375 4715
info@ampainsoc.org
www.ampainsoc.org

American Society for Pain Management Nursing
PO Box 15473
Lenexa, KS 66285-5473
Tel: +1 913 752 4975
aspmn@goamp.com
www.aspmn.org

American Society of Regional Anesthesia and Pain Medicine
520 N Northwest Highway
Park Ridge, IL 60068-2573
Tel: +1 847 825 7246
asra@asahq.org
www.asra.com

National Pain Education Council

c/o CME Scholar
1010 Washington Blvd., 7th Floor
Stamford, CT 06901
Tel: 1 888 536 7545
www.npecweb.org

The National Pain Foundation

300 E Hampden Avenue, Suite 100
Englewood, CO 80113
aardrup@nationalpainfoundation.org
www.nationalpainfoundation.org

NIH Pain Consortium

National Institutes of Health
Bethesda, MD 20892
braininfo@ninds.nih.gov
painconsortium.nih.gov

Partners Against Pain

One Stamford Forum
Stamford, CT 06901-3431
Tel: 1 888 726 7535
partnersagainstpain@pharma.com
www.partnersagainstpain.com

Trigeminal Neuralgia Association

925 Northwest 56th Terrace
Suite C, Gainesville, FL 32605-6402
Toll-free: 1 800 923 3608
Tel: +1 352 331 7009
tnational@tna-support.org
www.tna-support.org

International

Australian Pain Society

Suite 1, Ground Floor, 26 Ridge St
North Sydney NSW 2060
Tel: +61 (0)2 9954 4400
www.apsoc.org.au

Canadian Pain Society

701 Rossland Road East, Suite 373
Whitby, Ontario L1N 9K3
Tel: +1 905 668 9545
www.canadianpainsociety.ca

European Federation of IASP Chapters

Foukithidou 2
16343 Iliopoulis
Athens, Greece
Tel: +30 210 992 6335
efic@internet.gr
www.efic.org

European Society of Regional Anaesthesia and Pain Therapy

www.esraeurope.org

Faculty of Pain Medicine of the Australian and New Zealand College of Anaesthetists

'Ulimaroa', 630 St Kilda Road
Melbourne, Victoria 3004
Tel: +61 (0)3 9510 6299
painmed@anzca.edu.au
www.fpm.anzca.edu.au

International Association for the
Study of Pain
111 Queen Anne Ave. N, Suite 501
Seattle, WA 98109-4955
Tel: +1 206 283 0311
www.iasp-pain.org

International MYOPAIN Society
(Myofascial pain and
Fibromyalgia Syndrome)
c/o Ziemssenstrasse 1
D-80336 Munich, Germany
Tel: +49 (0)89 51 60 74 00
www.myopain.org

International Pelvic Pain Society
Tel: +1 847 517 8712
www.pelvicpain.org

NeuropathicPainNetwork
www.neuropathicpainnetwork.org

Pain South Africa
PO Box 12800
Amalinda 5252, East London
Tel/Fax: +27 (0)43 642 1928
painsouthafrica@iafrica.com
www.pain-management.co.za

Trigeminal Neuralgia Association
of Canada
1514 Lakemount Boulevard
South Lethbridge, Alberta T1K 3K4
Tel: +1 403 327 7668
president@tnac.org
www.tnac.org

Other useful resources
Australian National Health and
Medical Research Council
Acute pain management: scientific
evidence. 2nd edn. 2005.
www.nhmrc.gov.au/publications/
_files/cp104.pdf

Bandolier
Evidence-based thinking about
healthcare
www.jr2.ox.ac.uk/Bandolier

Medlineplus
www.nlm.nih.gov/medlineplus

Medicines and Healthcare
Products Regulatory Agency
Cardiovascular safety of NSAIDs:
review of evidence
www.mhra.gov.uk/home/idcplg?IdcS
ervice=GET_FILE&dDocName=con
1004303&RevisionSelectionMetho
d=Latest

Partners Against Pain
Pain assessment
www.partnersagainstpain.com/index
-mp.aspx?sid=3&aid=7824

Index